YEAST FREE LIFE

By
SARAH L. RHODES

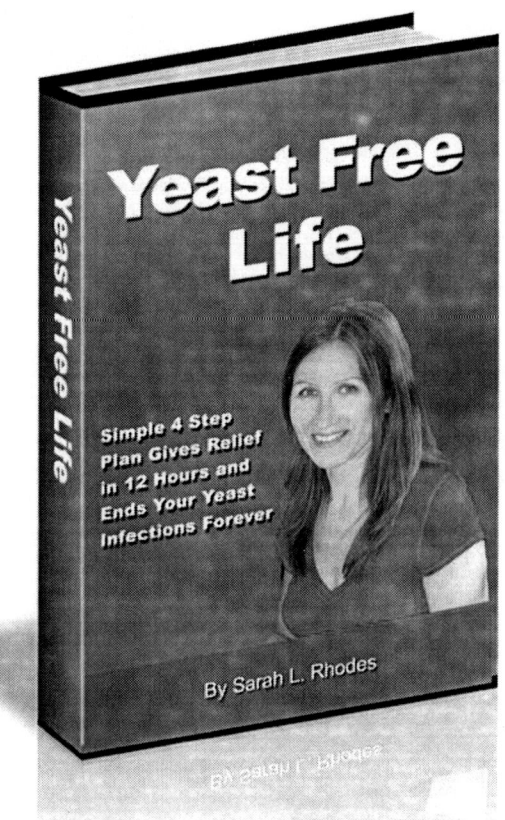

Copyright 2008 Sarah Rhodes YeastFreeLife.com
All rights reserved

DISCLAIMER

While all attempts have been made to verify information provided in this publication, neither the author nor the publisher assumes any responsibility for errors, omissions, or contrary interpretation of the subject matter herein. Any perceived slights of specific persons, peoples, or organizations are unintentional. The author neither makes nor attempts to make any diagnosis or cure or prevent any disease.

This is an informational product based on the experiences, research, and opinions of the author and is not intended as a source of medical advice. Information contained herein may be subject to varying national, state, and/or local laws or regulations.

The information in this product has not been evaluated by the FDA or anyone in the medical profession. It is not intended to replace advice and treatment from your medical practitioner or other qualified professional and it is not intended to be a substitute for professional medical care.

The author and publisher assume no responsibility or liability whatsoever on the behalf of any purchaser or reader of these materials.

You should consult your physician before applying any treatment or attempting anything mentioned in this book.

TABLE OF CONTENTS

1. INTRODUCTION **5**

2. WHAT IS YEAST INFECTION ? **9**

3. WHAT CAUSES YEAST INFECTION? **12**

    Compromised Immune System 12

    Hormones 16

    Diet 17

    Stress 17

    Loss of Our Helper Bacteria 18

4. DO I HAVE YEAST INFECTION? **21**

    Symptoms - **Acute Yeast Infection** 22

    Symptoms - Chronic Yeast Infection 24

    The Yeast Infection Test 29

5. 12 HOUR RELIEF TREATMENT **41**

    Vaginal Yeast Infections 42

    Skin Yeast Infection 49

    Yeast Infections of the Mouth and Throat (Thrush) 52

Yeast Infection of the Fingernails and Toenails 55

Yeast Infections of the Penis 57

6. YEAST FREE LIFE – THE PERMANENT CURE ... 62

Diet and Supplementation 67

The Die-Off Process 76

Kill Existing Candida Overgrowth 85

Internal Cleansing 87

Adding Friendly Bacteria 102

7. A FINAL WORD 108

APPENDIX 1 - CONVENTIONAL DRUGS AND TREATMENTS 110

1. INTRODUCTION

Hello,

I am Sarah Rhodes, the author of Yeast Free Life. I'd like to congratulate you on purchasing this book and your decision to take the first step toward having a completely Yeast Free Life. I know that sounds incredible right now and I don't blame you for having some doubts. After all, if you are like most people who arrive at this point you have been suffering and searching for quite awhile.

You may be one of thousands of women and men you are experiencing a wide and strange variety of symptoms ranging from mild rash and itching to horrible pain and discomfort. You may be experiencing these symptoms on the inside or the outside of your body...or maybe both. The symptoms may vary in intensity from mildly irritating to completely debilitating. Your symptoms may be constant or you may feel horrible one day and not-so-bad the next.

You may have arrived at this point already knowing that your symptoms are caused by yeast infection or, like so many others, you may still be searching for the cause of the symptoms that are negatively affecting your life in so many ways, great and small.

Regardless of what brought you here, you have made the right choice. I promise that in the pages that follow you will learn the simple steps for determining if you have a yeast infection, how to get rid of the immediate symptoms in as little as 12 hours, and how to completely eliminate yeast infections from your life...forever.

I know that is quite a promise and I don't make it lightly. In fact, I would not make it at all if I hadn't experienced the healing first-hand in my own life. I will never forget the pain, sick feeling, stress, and embarrassment that I felt when I suffered from yeast infections.

I tried over-the-counter medications that only gave me temporary relief at best. Then I went from doctor to doctor. The symptoms were sometimes hard to describe and it seemed that some doctors didn't take me seriously. Other doctors prescribed prescription medications. I remember thinking that surely these medications would solve my problems...but they didn't. In fact, some of the medications seemed to make things worse and, as I realized later, actually put my life in danger.

Unable to find permanent help I began 5 years of medical research, study, experimentation, and trial-and-error to develop a permanent cure for this horrible disease. I talked to doctors, nurses, nutritionists, naturopaths, and authors and I studied all of the medical literature I could find on the subject.

I guess I'd have to admit that finding this cure became a bit of an obsession with me. But, I was still suffering with the symptoms of yeast infections and I knew that millions of others were too so I was very motivated.

The more I studied, the more I realized that the doctors and the pharmaceutical companies have it all wrong. They are totally focused on treating the symptoms of the disease but are completely ignoring its root causes. This was the revelation that resulted in the step-by-step plan contained in this book.

I followed these steps, made the adjustments that I needed to make in my life, got my body in balance, and I can now say that I now have a permanent, total, and complete Yeast Free Life. Even better, I have shared this plan with thousands of women and men throughout the world and have thrilled at the emails I have received telling me how their lives have been changed simply by following this plan.

That is why I can promise you that your life will be changed. I have experienced tremendous changes in my own life and I have seen and heard about the countless lives that have been changed by this plan.

It is my greatest desire that you will find healing and peace in the words of this book.

2. WHAT IS YEAST INFECTION?

Before we can begin to talk about curing our yeast infections we need to have a basic understanding of what a yeast infection is. I know you are reading this book because you or someone you care about suffers from yeast infections. You probably don't care a lot about the medical terminology or detailed scientific explanations so I'll try not to burden you with either. There are plenty of books and websites that will make this sound very complicated. The truth is that the whole subject is just not that complicated and the remedy is pretty simple. What follows is the simple explanation that I believe you need to know to get started on the path to a permanent cure.

What we commonly call a "yeast infection" is actually a mold infection that occurs when there is an overgrowth of yeast organisms within our body. By far the most common yeast is called Candida (pronounced Can-DEE-da).

Candida is actually helpful to our bodies and it occurs naturally in or on the vagina, mouth, throat, skin and digestive tract. When our bodies are properly balanced Candida does not cause any problems. Our body's defenses and helper bacteria keep the yeast under control. Only when conditions are not right within the body can it grow out of control and cause an infection.

Candida exists in two forms…yeast and mold. In its yeast form Candida is helpful to our bodies…or, at the very least, not harmful. Our problems start when Candida changes from its yeast form to its mold form. This happens when conditions within our bodies get out of balance. This out-of-balance condition allows the yeast to multiply rapidly and turn into mold and that is what is commonly called a "yeast infection."

When the yeast form of Candida turns into mold some very bad things begin to happen:

First, the mold sends out long hook-like legs. These hooks dig into membranes throughout the body and burrow between our skin cells.

Second, the mold attacks our cells by secreting enzymes that break down the cell walls and allow the mold to absorb the nutrients from the cells.

Third, our body responds to this invasion like it does to any other infection...with swelling, heat, and pain. White blood cells, antibodies, and other factors in the blood collect at the site of the invasion and attack the invading mold.

Fourth, if unchecked, the hook-like legs can grow through the mucous membranes of the intestinal tract and allow toxins from the intestines to pass directly into the bloodstream and spread throughout the body. This is the cause of many elusive symptoms that we experience when we have a yeast infection. We will talk more about symptoms later.

That is my simple, straight forward explanation of what a yeast infection is. I know the thought of having these hook-like legs growing inside and attacking our cells is a pretty scary thing...and, it should be! We are all too familiar with the pain and discomfort these attacks can cause and, if left untreated, the infection can become systemic and life threatening.

Now that we know what a yeast infection is, let's discuss its causes.

3. WHAT CAUSES YEAST INFECTION?

Candida always lives with us and only becomes a problem when it grows out of control. Usually, our body's natural defenses protect us. When these defenses break down our bodies get out of balance, the yeast has an opportunity to multiply rapidly and change to mold, and we have a yeast infection. Following are the factors that most often contribute to a Candida overgrowth. Each factor can cause damage to the body's defenses. Several factors in combination can mount a serious attack on the body.

Compromised Immune System

A compromised immune system is probably the largest general cause of yeast infections. Doctors know that the weaker our immune system is, the more likely we are to develop a yeast infection. A weakened immune system can stem from a variety of factors, the most common being the prolonged use of antibiotics.

Antibiotics fight off infections by killing bacteria. Unfortunately, most antibiotics not only kill the bad bacteria that cause illness but they also kill the good (helper) bacteria that keep Candida under control and prevent it from turning into mold. Without the helper bacteria yeast is left to grow without restriction in the body. Antibiotics change the environment of the gut, so that our helper bacteria can't protect us from Candida overgrowth and other harmful organisms.

Yeast expert Dr. William Crook, in his book The Yeast Connection, says, "Many different factors play a part in making you sick, yet I am convinced that repeated courses of broad-spectrum antibiotics are the main 'villain'. These antibiotics cause yeast overgrowth in your intestinal tract and vaginal yeast infections. And these infections, like a stream cascading down a mountain, set off disturbances which can make you feel 'sick all over'.

Doctors also realize that chronic yeast infections can occur in people who have extremely compromised immune systems, such as diabetics and those with immune dysfunction disorders. Again, the same concept can apply to people whose immune systems are otherwise normal, but have other factors which, when added together, lead to an unhealthy immune system.

Most people are surprised to learn that they may be taking antibiotics without even knowing it. We are exposed to antibiotics when we eat dairy and meat products because farm animals are often given antibiotics to stimulate growth and to treat infections. Just as if we were taking the antibiotics directly, constant exposure to antibiotics through the food we eat kills the susceptible bacteria and leaves behind more resistant forms of bacteria. Unfortunately, Pasteurization or cooking can't kill or remove antibiotics in our food.

Many people who report symptoms of yeast infection have suffered from a recent illness or have a long history of use of antibiotics, birth control pills, or steroids. Finally, the body has had enough. For these people, even though there is no single "big" reason for yeast infection to start, there are a lot of smaller reasons that pile up.

When just the right (or should I say "wrong") combination of conditions occurs in our bodies the Candida can take advantage of our weak immune systems and the unfortunate overgrowth process begins.

Anything that interferes with the body's normal immune system can lead to an overgrowth of yeast in the body. Some of these interfering factors are:

- Repeated or prolonged use of antibiotics
- Prolonged use of prednisone or other steroid medications
- Vitamin/mineral/nutrient deficiencies
- Use of birth control pills
- Hormonal changes
- Alcohol use
- Excessive stress
- Hormone Replacement Therapy
- Use of immunosuppressive medications
- Pregnancy
- Immune dysfunction disorders
- Diabetes
- Cancer treatments
- Chemical poisoning from home or workplace substances
- Thyroid disease
- AIDS

These factors (particularly the use of antibiotics) can temporarily lower the body's immune system long enough for Candida to take hold and begin to grow rapidly. Once this has begun, the symptoms may appear quickly, or develop slowly over time.

Remember, though, that it is not just the amount of yeast that exists that causes the problems. The bigger problem is caused when the yeast converts to mold which causes more damage and releases toxins into the body. These toxins cause even more damage and further weaken the immune system. Once this destructive cycle begins it can only be totally stopped by bringing the body's systems back into balance.

Hormones

Birth control pills and Hormone Replacement Therapy (HRT) can contribute to Candida overgrowth. Candida loves grows rapidly in the presence of progesterone, which is found in the birth control pills and HRT.

Many women find an increase in yeast infection symptoms during the week before your menstrual period, when progesterone levels are highest and hormones are causing a change in the vaginal environment. Often the vaginal membranes are unable to defend against invading yeast because of nutritional deficiencies, possibly as a result of taking the birth control pill.

Diet

We will talk much more about diet later in the book but, for now, I will simply say that Candida thrives on sugar. A high sugar diet is a recipe for yeast infections. With all of the junk food and high sugar content foods that most of us eat our bodies are absorbing massive amounts of sugar and providing Candida with a constant over-supply of food. I will have a lot more to say about what to eat and what not eat in a later chapter.

Stress

Scientists now realize that stress affects the body both emotionally and physically. When we are under stress, our bodies produce chemicals that weaken our immune system. This doesn't just apply to people who have trouble handling stress or who "stress out" often. Our immune system is affected by stress even if we appear to handle it well.

Stress also changes the bacterial environment in our gut, interrupting the balance our helper bacteria. This change in bacteria can allow Candida to take over and multiply. As it rapidly grows Candida turns against our body by creating its toxins to fight the helper bacteria thus compromising our immune system. Once the body's defenses are weakened, Candida takes control and usually wins the battle.

Loss of Our Helper Bacteria

When I refer to the "gut" I am talking about inside of the intestinal tract. It is a muscular tube that breaks down food and extracts the nutrients. The leftover matter is then deposited as waste (feces). "Friendly" helper bacteria help keep our gut safe from dangerous viruses, bacteria, yeast, and parasites. These bacteria help us digest our food and provide us with some nutrients.

Most of what we hear about bacteria is negative. If we listen to the pharmaceutical companies we would think that we should be doing everything we can to kill all of the bacteria in our bodies. Surprisingly, the average person has over 400 species of bacteria living in their gut, from mouth to anus. The bacteria in the large intestine weigh about three pounds. These bacteria are essential to our health and wellbeing.

These helper bacteria help in digestion by breaking down sugar, fats, carbohydrates, and protein. Helper bacteria also keep the intestine acidic, which helps control the growth of Candida. A healthy body requires a healthy gut and a healthy gut requires healthy helper bacteria.

When our gut is healthy, Candida is naturally kept in balance. Our helper bacteria compete with Candida yeast for nutrients and sugars and keep it under control. Reducing the level of helper bacteria through the prolonged or frequent use of antibiotics upsets the balance and allows Candida to take control.

Whatever is in your stomach goes into your small intestine and on into your large intestine. If you take an antibiotic capsule, the drug will end up in your large intestine where it will destroy bacteria. Destroying bacteria is what antibiotics are supposed to do. However, when the helper bacteria are destroyed, the gut's main defense is destroyed. Candida can take over. It can grow and infect our cells and cause them to die.

Antibiotics can kill bacteria but they cannot kill yeast. Through prolonged use of antibiotics the helper bacteria are killed and the yeast is allowed to grow uncontrolled. Eventually Candida changes from its yeast form into its dangerous mold form and starts destroying cells. This also interferes with our digestion and weakens our metabolism.

When the gut's environment changes, whether from the birth control pills, antibiotics, or other drugs, or when you are experiencing a high level of stress, combined with sugar or alcohol, Candida thrives and can grow into a full blown yeast infection.

4. DO I HAVE YEAST INFECTION?

Now that we understand what a yeast infection is and some of the factors that can cause it, let's start getting personal. Before we proceed to discuss treatment alternatives we must first answer the obvious question…"Do I have a yeast infection?" First we will discuss some of the symptoms of acute and chronic yeast infections and then we will go right into the test with which we will see, with a high degree of certainty whether or not you are experiencing a yeast infection.

Yeast infections fall into two categories…Acute and Chronic.

With acute yeast infections the symptoms develop rapidly and are generally localized. Localized vaginal infection and oral thrush are examples of acute yeast infections. If we can treat the infection successfully at this stage, the symptoms and the infection may go away.

Chronic yeast infections occur when the roots of the fungus really take hold, so that you are infected deep into your tissues. This is the stage of the infection that stays with us over a long period of time.

Symptoms of Acute Yeast Infection

Symptoms of acute yeast infections vary with the location of the infection and include:

Skin:

Rash, itchiness, soreness, flakiness, white patches, redness

Skin folds:

Rash, itchiness, soreness, flakiness, white patches, redness, weeping sores

Nails:

Discoloration, ridges, brittleness, abnormal thickening, fragile nails, flaking

Mouth:

White patches, bad breath, pain, cracks at the corner of the mouth

Esophagus:

Pain on swallowing, heartburn, cough, sore throat

Intestinal Tract:

Indigestion, gas, bloating, food intolerance, constipation, blood in stool, diarrhea

Anal Area:

Pain, itchiness, burning on bowel movements, weeping sores

Vagina/Vulva:

Itchiness, pain, redness, "cottage cheese" discharge, painful and/or frequent urination, swollen glands, painful intercourse

Penis:

Itchiness, redness, white spots, pain on urination, white discharge from the end of the penis

Bladder:

Painful and/or frequent urination, blood in urine

Symptoms of Chronic Yeast Infection

While the symptoms of acute yeast infections are usually confined to the infected area, chronic yeast infections can show up throughout the body in many areas at the same time.

Candida can take root in any body tissue. It can live in your bones and joints as well as the tissues of the heart, kidney, liver, brain, and muscle. Once the infection takes root it causes inflammation in that tissue. The effects of that inflammation are widely varied depending upon where the infection has taken root.

Chronic Candida overgrowth can cause so many different symptoms that it is almost impossible to exclude any symptom. Symptoms often change over time as our bodies fight the infection in one area only to have it reemerge in a completely different area. The severity of the symptoms can also change over time. Because of this, many of us have gone undiagnosed and untreated by our health care professional for years.

Symptoms may stay steady and predictable for awhile and then change rapidly overnight. We may have severe symptoms one day and only mild symptoms or even no symptoms at all the next day. A common complaint for yeast infection sufferers is having a vague feeling of being unwell all the time....not quite sick but definitely not well. Others with chronic yeast infections may be so ill that they can't get out of bed or function in their daily lives.

People with a chronic yeast infection usually exhibit some or all of the following symptoms:

- Feeling generally unwell
- Fatigue
- Muscle and joint aches and pains
- Lack of energy
- Mood changes
- Weight change
- Stomach and bowel problems

Because the Candida overgrowth can attack anywhere in the body and in multiple places at the same time there is an almost endless list of other symptoms that it can cause. They include:

- Poor memory
- Joint pain
- Moodiness
- PMS
- Poor concentration
- Lack of energy
- Chronic tiredness
- Irritability
- Cough
- Pneumonia
- Hyperactivity
- Allergies
- Altered or poor sleep
- Lack of interest in sex
- Relationship problems
- Mood swings
- Abdominal pain
- Diarrhea
- Urinary tract infection
- Brain infection
- Heart Infection
- Liver infection
- Bone infection
- Ulcers
- Gas and bloating
- Flatulence
- Depression

- Muscle pain
- Endometriosis
- Skin infection
- Eye infection
- Penis infection
- Vaginal infection
- Endocrine, hormonal imbalance
- Dry skin, itching
- Bladder infection
- Eye infection, burning eyes
- Food cravings
- Heartburn
- Frequent sore throats
- Frequent infections
- Asthma
- Premature skin aging
- Weight loss and weight gain
- Bad breath

Chances are high that you are experiencing some, or even many, of these symptoms. If you see some familiar symptoms in the lists above there is a good possibility you have a yeast infection.

To help determine with a high degree of certainty that your symptoms are, in fact, being caused by yeast infection I have included a comprehensive test on the next few pages.

This test is divided into 3 sections...A, B, and C. Just answer the questions honestly and add up the points for each section. Then add your scores for the 3 sections together to determine how likely it is that your symptoms are being caused by yeast infection.

THE YEAST INFECTION TEST

SECTION A: History

1. Have you ever taken acne medication for 1 month or longer?
    _____ Yes (35 points)
    _____ No (0 points)

2. Have you ever taken broad spectrum antibiotics or other antibacterial medication for respiratory, urinary, or other infections for 2 months or longer or for shorter periods 4 or more times in a 1 year period?
    _____ Yes (35 points)
    _____ No (0 points)

3. Have you ever taken a broad-spectrum antibiotic drug – even in a single does?
    _____ Yes (6 points)
    _____ No (0 points)

4. Have you ever been bothered by persistent prostatitis, vaginitis, or other

problems affecting your reproductive organs?
_____ Yes (25 points)
_____ No (0 points)

5. Are you bothered by memory or concentration problems – do you sometimes feel spaced out?
_____ Yes (20 points)
_____ No (0 points)

6. Do you feel "sick all over" yet, in spite of visits to many different physicians, the causes haven't been found?
_____ Yes (20 points)
_____ No (0 points)

7. How many times have you been pregnant?
_____ 2 or more times (5 points)
_____ 1 time (3 points)
_____ Never (0 points)

8. How long have you taken birth control pills?
_____ more than 2 years (15 points)

_____ 6 month to 2 years
(8 points)
_____ less then 6 months or
never   (0 points)

9. Have you taken steroids orally, by injection, or inhalation...
_____ for more than 2 weeks? (15 points)
_____ 2 weeks or less? (6 points)

10. Does exposure to perfumes, insecticides, fabric shop odors, and other chemicals provoke moderate to severe symptoms?
_____ Yes (20 points)

Only mild symptoms?
_____ Yes (5 points)

No symptoms?
_____ Yes (0 points)

11. Does tobacco smoke really bother you?
_____ Yes (10 points)
_____ No (0 points)

12. Are your symptoms worse on damp, muggy days or in moldy places?
　　_____ Yes (20 points)
　　_____ No (0 points)

13. If you have you had athlete's foot, ring work, "jock itch" or other chronic fungus infections of the skin or nails have such infections been:

Severe or Persistent?
　　_____ Yes (20 points)

Mild to moderate?
　　_____ Yes (10 points)

None?
　　_____ Yes (0 points)

14. Do you crave sugar?
　　_____ Yes (10 points)
　　_____ No (0 points)

TOTAL POINTS for Section A: _____

SECTION B: Major Symptoms

For each of your symptoms, enter the appropriate figure in the Point Score column:

If a symptom is occasional or mild…………………..……….3 points
If a symptom is frequent and/or moderately severe…….6 points
If a symptom is severe and/or disabling…………………..9 points

Add the total score and record at the end of this section.

1. _____   Fatigue or lethargy

2. _____   Feeling of being "drained"

3. _____   Depression or manic depression

4. _____   Numbness, burning or tingling

5. _____   Headache

6. _____ Muscle aches

7. _____ Muscle weakness or paralysis

8. _____ Pain and/or swelling in joints

9. _____ Abdominal pain

10. _____ Constipation and/or diarrhea

11. _____ Bloating, belching, or intestinal gas

12. _____ Troublesome vaginal burning, itching, or discharge

13. _____ Prostatitis

14. _____ Impotence

15. _____ Loss of sexual desire or feeling

16. _____ Endometriosis or infertility

17. _____ Cramps and/or other menstrual irregularities

18. _____ Premenstrual tension

19. _____ Attacks of anxiety or crying

20. _____ Cold hands or feet, low body temperature

21. _____ Hypothyroidism

22. _____ Shaking or irritable when hungry

23. _____ Cystitis or interstitial cystitis

TOTAL SCORE for Section B: _____

Section C: Other Symptoms

For each of your symptoms, enter the appropriate figure in the Point Score column:

If a symptom is occasional or mild…………………..………….1 points

If a symptom is frequent and/or moderately severe……..2 points

If a symptom is severe and/or disabling…………………....…3 points

Add the total score and record at the end of this section.

1. _____   Drowsiness

2. _____   Irritability

3. _____   Lack of coordination

4. _____   Frequent mood swings

5. _____   Insomnia

6. _____   Dizziness/loss of balance

7. _____ Pressure above the ears...feeling of head swelling

8. _____ Sinus problems...tenderness of cheekbones or forehead

9. _____ Tendency to bruise easily

10. _____ Eczema, itching eyes

11. _____ Psoriasis

12. _____ Chronic hives

13. _____ Indigestion or heartburn

14. _____ Sensitivity to milk, wheat, corn, or other common foods.

15. _____ Mucus in stools

16. _____ Rectal itching

17. _____ Dry mouth or throat

18. _____ Mouth rashes, including white tongue

19. _____ Bad breath

20. _____ Foot, hair, or body odor not relieved by washing

21. _____ Nasal congestion or postnasal drip

22. _____ Nasal itching

23. _____ Sore throat

24. _____ Laryngitis, loss of voice

25. _____ Cough or recurrent bronchitis

26. _____ Pain or tightness in chest

27. _____ Wheezing or shortness of breath

28. _____ Urinary frequency or urgency

29. _____ Burning on urination

30. _____ Spots in front of eyes or erratic vision

31. _____ Burning or tearing eyes

32. _____ Recurrent infection or fluid in ears

33. _____ Ear pain or deafness

TOTAL SCORE, Section C: _____

Total Score for Section A: _____
Total Score for Section B: _____
Total Score for Section C: _____

GRAND TOTAL SCORE: _____

The Grand Total Score will help you decide if your health problems are yeast-connected. Scores in women will run higher, as seven items in the questionnaire apply exclusively to women, while only two apply exclusively to men.

Yeast-connected health problems are almost certainly present in women with scores higher than 180 and in men with scores higher than 140.

Yeast-connected health problems are probably present in women with scores higher than 120 and in men with scores higher than 90.

Yeast-connected health problems are possibly present in women with scores higher than 60 and in men with scores higher than 40.

With scores less than 60 in women and 40 in men, yeasts are less likely to cause health problems.

5. 12 HOUR RELIEF TREATMENT

If you currently have an acute yeast infection your main goal right now is to get rid of the symptoms. Before we can start working on your yeast free life we must stop the itching, inflammation, burning, and swelling you are now experiencing.

Fortunately, there are some easy, safe, simple, and 100% natural ways to eliminate those annoying symptoms...usually in less than 12 hours. Better yet, the ingredients you need are cheap and may be in your refrigerator already. If not, you can get them at the local market or health foods store.

For obvious reasons, the 12 hour relief treatment method varies depending upon where on your body the yeast infection is. I have separated the treatments into 5 areas depending on where your symptoms are occurring. They are yeast infections of the (a) vagina, (b) skin, (c) mouth/throat, (d) nails, and (e) penis.

Vaginal Yeast Infections

Symptoms of Vaginal Yeast Infection

We will discuss yeast infections of the vagina first because it is the most common. About 75% of all women will get at least one vaginal yeast infection in their lifetime.

The first sign of a vaginal yeast infection is usually an odorless discharge that looks like cottage cheese. Vaginal discharge is not always present and if it is it may be so slight that you may not even notice it. The severity of other symptoms may vary from quite mild to severe. You may even have no symptoms at all. If you have never had a yeast infection before please see a health care professional before starting any treatment so that you can be sure you do not have a more serious condition.

The most common symptoms of a vaginal yeast infection are:

(1) Vaginal burning.
(2) Vaginal itching.
(3) Vulva irritation
(4) White, cheesy discharge or thick whitish-gray discharge that may have an odor like baking yeast.

(5) Redness, swelling, and discharge from the mucous membranes of the vagina.
(6) Discomfort during or after sexual intercourse.
(7) Inflammation, swelling, or burning of the external vaginal area (the vulva).
(8) Painful urination
(9) Frequent urination.

Natural Treatment for Vaginal Yeast Infections

The natural 12 hour treatment for vaginal yeast infections is done in 3 steps. Step 1 uses garlic inserted into the vagina to kill the yeast overgrowth, step 2 is an apple cider vinegar douche that restores the pH balance in the vagina to make it hard for the yeast to regrow, and step 3 uses a yogurt tampon to reintroduce friendly bacteria to the vagina.

Step 1 - Garlic Tampons

Garlic has, among its many health benefits, a strong antimicrobial activity against various types of bacteria and fungi. When applied to an area where yeast infection is present it can quickly and effectively kill the yeast and eliminate the symptoms of infection. For a vaginal yeast infection we need to get the garlic into the vagina using the following method:

Peel a garlic clove. Be careful not to nick it, as some women find the garlic oil can burn. You might feel a slight burning sensation for the first few minutes but that should go away quickly. Wrap the clove in a thin piece of cheese cloth or gauze, fold the cloth in half and tie a knot, leaving some extra at the end, or just twist the cloth into a tail. Insert it in the vagina like a tampon. Alternatively, you can insert the garlic without the cloth. Remove the clove by inserting a finger behind the clove and popping it out like a diaphragm. Replace the tampon with a fresh garlic clove every 2 to 4 hours. Continue this process for a total of 10 to 12 hours.

Step 2 - Apple Cider Vinegar Douche

The apple cider vinegar douche is performed after using the garlic tampon treatment for at least 12 hours. The garlic should have killed most of the yeast overgrowth and your symptoms should be about gone. Now it is time to change the environment of the vagina to make it hard for the yeast to regrow.

Apple cider vinegar is a powerful antiseptic and antibiotic. I suggest you use only raw, unfiltered apple cider made from organic apples. The vinegar acts as a powerful cleanser and will help adjust the acid-alkaline balance, which creates an environment in which yeast cannot grow. Using apple cider vinegar as a douche will quickly restore the natural pH of the vagina and eliminate the remaining yeast overgrowth.

Prepare a solution with 2 tablespoons of apple cider vinegar per 1 quart of lukewarm (not hot) water. Fill a douche bag with the solution and apply to the vagina. Be careful to keep the bag below your pelvis and only exert slight pressure. Move the nozzle slowly to prevent damage to your vaginal walls. I have found the most effective way to apply the douche is lying on my side on a towel in an empty bathtub.

If you prefer, you can use a meat baster instead of a douche bag or soak a small natural sponge in the solution, insert it into your vagina and leave it for several hours.

Step 3 – Yogurt Tampon

Yogurt contains friendly probiotic bacteria such as acidophilus and bifidus that defend against the overgrowth of yeast. Most commercial brands of yogurt are heated to increase the shelf life and they contain few or no friendly bacteria. Even if the yogurt package says "made with active cultures" the cultures may have been destroyed in the manufacturing process.

Be sure to use yogurt that is plain (unflavored) and that contains no sugar, additives, or coloring and that has not been heat treated. You will be able to find what you need in most health food stores.

For this step you can use a regular tampon dipped into the yogurt or you can simply squirt the yogurt into your vagina with a syringe (with the needle removed). Most women find it easiest to simply dip a tampon into the yogurt and insert it into the vagina in the usual way.

You should feel an immediate cooling and soothing sensation. Leave the yogurt in place for about 1 hour.

Following these 3 steps will eliminate the symptoms for 90% of women who are suffering from a vaginal yeast infection. If your infection is particularly severe and you are still having symptoms after the 12 hour treatment you should perform all 3 steps again.

By now the symptoms of your vaginal yeast infection should be gone. Please understand that we have not eliminated yeast infections from your life. So far we have only given you relief from the immediate attack you were experiencing. We will learn how to achieve the yeast free life in the next chapter.

Prevention of Vaginal Yeast Infections.

There are a few things I recommend doing to help keep prevent future vaginal yeast infections:

1. Do not wear clothing that fits tight in your crotch. If you wear panty hose only wear the kind that have a cotton crotch panel. Only wear cotton underwear. Yeast infections are 3 times more likely to occur with women who wear nylon underwear than with those who wear

cotton underwear. Cotton allows the vagina to "breathe."

2. Avoid wearing damp clothing, including bathing suits, for any extended periods of time.

3. Be sure to dry your outer vaginal area completely after bathing because a warm, moist environment encourages yeast to grow.

4. Do not douche, except for the natural douche treatments outlined in this book. Douches rinse away healthy vaginal secretions and friendly bacteria and can also cause the surface of the vaginal area to become too dry.

5. Do not use perfumed feminine hygiene sprays.

6. Avoid bubble baths and non-organic soaps. Soap is a harsh alkaline (especially brand name, chemical ones), and it upsets the normal pH of your vagina. Most bubble baths are detergents that may break down the protective barrier that vaginal bacteria offer against infection.

Skin Yeast Infection

Symptoms of Yeast Infection of the Skin

Yeast infections of the skin commonly occur in warm moist body areas, such as underarms. Usually, the skin effectively blocks yeast, but any breakdown or cuts in the skin may allow the organism to penetrate and cause an infection. The warm moist areas such as in skin folds, arm pits, below the breasts, upper thighs, and groin/anal areas provide a friendly environment for yeast to grow and are the most common areas of the skin to become infected.

Yeast infections of the skin are usually seen as a local rash, usually red with swelling. The rash is usually well defined from the surrounding skin and has a sharp border. The area often becomes itchy and has a clear odorless discharge. If the infection exists for a long time, the skin can thicken and become scaly.

Natural Treatments for Yeast Infections of the Skin

Treat the symptoms of skin yeast infections with a 3 step process:

Step 1 – Raw Honey

Raw honey has some amazing antibacterial, antiviral, and antibiotic properties. It is a powerful antioxidant and has a powerful ability to heal wounds and treat yeast infections. Try to find raw, pure, unheated, and unprocessed honey.

Take a generous portion of honey in your hand and spread it over the infected area. Keep the area saturated with honey for at least 10 minutes. Rinse the area with warm water to remove the honey and gently pat dry. Do not rub because you might do further damage to the skin. You should feel relief almost instantly after applying the honey.

Step 2 – Apple Cider Vinegar Soak

Prepare a solution of 4 tablespoons of apple cider vinegar to 1 quart of warm water. We will now soak the infected area in the solution for 20 minutes to kill any remaining yeast and restore the natural pH to the skin. Depending upon where the infection in located you might need to soak a natural sponge or cotton cloth in the solution and hold it on the area.

Step 3 – Yogurt

Now we will restore the good bacteria to the skin by applying plain (unflavored) yogurt that contains no sugar, additives, coloring, and that has not been heat treated. We want yogurt that has active, living, probiotics such as acidophilus and bifidus.

Spread the yogurt evenly over the infected area with your fingers. Leave the area with the yogurt for 1 hour.

After following these 3 steps the yeast infection should be gone and the symptoms should be significantly reduced. It may take a few days for the skin to completely heal from the infection. There are a few more steps you can take to help the healing process:

1. Keep the area dry.
2. If the infected area is in your arm pits, avoid using deodorant for at least 3 days.
3. Do not use cornstarch. If you need to use powder, use only unscented talc.
4. Apply Tea Tree Oil to the area twice daily for a week.

Tea Tree Oil is available at many health stores and online. I recommend Tea Tree Oil by Natures Sunshine which is can be purchased at:

http://NaturalLifeSuperstore.com/teatreeoil.html

5. Apply Oregano Oil to the area twice daily for a week. You can purchase Oregano Oil at some health stores or you can order a very powerful and pure Oregano Oil product at this site:

http://NaturalLifeSuperstore.com/oreganooil.html

Prevention of Skin Yeast Infection

There are a few simple things I recommend to avoid future skin yeast infections:

1. Keep infection-prone areas as dry as possible.
2. Wear loose clothing.
3. Do not wear wet clothing.

Yeast Infections of the Mouth and Throat (Thrush)

Symptoms of Mouth and Throat Yeast Infections

Yeast infection of the mouth and throat are characterized by white patches on the tongue, inner lips, and roof of the mouth which are often accompanied by mild to moderate pain. The white patches are not always visible when the infection is in the throat. The white patches may bleed slightly if you rub them or disturb them while brushing your teeth. As the infection progresses the patches may spread to the gums, throat, and tonsils.

Yeasts are part of the normal flora in the mouth. They ordinarily do not cause symptoms. Certain conditions, such as antibiotic use, can disturb the natural balance of microorganisms in the mouth and allow the overgrowth of Candida to cause thrush. Tetracycline and other broad-spectrum antibiotics frequently kill the good bacteria in the mouth, allowing the overgrowth of yeast.

Thrush is usually a minor and easily addressed problem, but it can be more serious for those with immune system disorders, such as AIDS.

Natural Treatment of Yeast Infections of the Mouth and Throat

Follow this 3 step process to eliminate the symptoms of yeast infections of the mouth and throat:

Step 1 – Garlic Rinse

Crush 1 garlic clove and mix it with 1 tablespoon of olive oil. Swish the mixture in your mouth, making contact as much as possible with the infected areas, for 5 minutes. The taste can be unpleasant for some and 5 minutes can seem like a very long time. Just do your best but don't be too concerned if you cannot do this for the entire 5 minutes.

Step 2 – Apple Cider Vinegar Rinse

This step will restore the pH balance in your mouth and throat and make it hard for the Candida to grow. Mix a solution of 2 tablespoons of apple cider vinegar with 1 cup of water. Rinse and gargle with the solution until it is all gone.

Step 3 – Yogurt Rinse

For most people the yogurt rinse is much more pleasant than the garlic rinse. All you need to do for this step is place about one tablespoon of plain (unflavored) live culture yogurt that contains no sugar, additives, coloring, and that has not been heat treated into your mouth and swish it around for 5 minutes.

Yeast Infection of the Fingernails and Toenails

Symptoms of Yeast Infections of the Nails

Yeast infections frequently occur on the skin around the base and sides of the nails. The infection can occur on both the hands and feet. People whose hands or feet are constantly wet are most susceptible to this infection. The skin at the base of the nail becomes red and painful over the period of a day or so. Occasionally, there is pus discharged from the sides of the nails. If the infection persists, the skin below the nail can become infected. If this occurs, the nail can become irregular, thickened and brittle, with ridges and groves in it.

Natural Treatment of Yeast Infection the Nails

The most successful method of treating infections in the skin around the edge of the nail is by applying Tea Tree Oil to the infected area. The Tea Tree Oil that I use and highly recommend is available at this site:

http://NaturalLifeSuperstore.com/teatreeoil.html

This oil should be applied twice daily and massaged into the affected area until the infection goes away.

When the yeast infection spreads under the nail, it becomes much more difficult to treat. This is because the area is protected by the nail surface. If Tea Tree Oil applied around and as far as possible under the nail does not eliminate the infection, treatment by a physician may be necessary.

Prevention of Yeast Infection of the Nails

There are a few simple things I recommend to avoid future nail infections:

1. Keep the hands and feet as dry as possible.
2. If your hands must be frequently immersed in water, protect your hands, nails and cuticles with lanolin, or wear gloves.
3. If you are prone to getting yeast infection under or around the nail, massage the nail and cuticle areas with Tea Tree Oil prior to prolonged exposure to water.

Yeast Infections of the Penis

Yeast infections in men are so hard to detect that most men will go throughout their entire lives without ever knowing that they have one. Men experience different symptoms than women typically do and their symptoms are not as noticeable. It is usually not until the infection causes other issues with their health that they take notice that something is wrong. Men can contract a yeast infection through intercourse when the man's urethra is exposed to the fungus which travels up the urethral canal to the prostate gland. Likewise, a man can transmit the infection to his sexual partner during intercourse.

Symptoms of Yeast Infections of the Penis

The signs of a male yeast infection include redness, itching and soreness of the penis, especially the head of the penis. Sometimes tiny red and itchy blisters may be present. It is possible that a white, cheesy discharge may present itself, often with an accompanying odor. Some of these signs may also indicate a sexually transmitted disease, so it is recommended that if treatment for the yeast infection does not work, a doctor should be seen immediately.

Male yeast infection symptoms are very similar to the symptoms experienced by women who have a vaginal yeast infection.

Here are some additional symptoms of male yeast:

1. Burning sensation when urinating

2. Pain during sexual intercourse
3. Rash (along the shaft or on the tip of the penis)
4. Burning sensation of the infected area
5. Slight swelling of the infected area
6. Light discharge

Natural Treatment for Yeast Infection of the Penis

Step 1 – Raw Honey

Raw honey has some amazing antibacterial, antiviral, and antibiotic properties. It is a powerful antioxidant and has a powerful ability to heal wounds and treat yeast infections. Try to find raw, pure, unheated, and unprocessed honey.

Take a generous portion of honey in your hand and spread it over the infected area. Keep the area saturated with honey for at least 10 minutes. Rinse the area with warm water to remove the honey and gently pat dry. Do not rub because you might do further damage to the skin. You should feel relief almost instantly after applying the honey.

Step 2 – Apple Cider Vinegar Soak

Prepare a solution of 4 tablespoons of apple cider vinegar to 1 quart of warm water. We will now soak the infected area in the solution for 20 minutes to kill any remaining yeast and restore the natural pH to the skin. Depending upon where the infection in located you might need to soak a natural sponge or cotton cloth in the solution and hold it on the area.

Step 3 – Yogurt

Now we will restore the good bacteria to the skin by applying plain (unflavored) yogurt that contains no sugar, additives, coloring, and that has not been heat treated. We want yogurt that has active, living, probiotics such as acidophilus and bifidus.

Spread the yogurt evenly over the infected area with your fingers. Leave the area with the yogurt for 1 hour.

Prevention of Yeast Infection of the Penis

Yeast infection frequently occurs in genitals where skin rubs against skin. It is important that your sexual partner be treated as the infection can be passed through sexual contact. You also should:

1. Keep the area dry and clean.
2. Avoid wearing wet clothing, such as bathing suits.
3. Wear loose underwear and loose clothing.
4. If using body powder, choose one containing unscented talc, not cornstarch.
5. To prevent infection from a sexual partner, use a condom.

6. YEAST FREE LIFE – THE PERMANENT CURE

If you stayed with me through the earlier chapters you now have a pretty good idea about what yeast infection is and what causes it. If you reviewed the long list of symptoms and took the test you can be very certain whether yeast overgrowth is causing your health problems. Hopefully, if you have a current acute yeast infection you have been able to apply the steps described in the previous chapter to reduce or eliminate your immediate symptoms.

It is now time to learn how to change your life permanently. What follows in this chapter is a step-by-step system for permanently removing yeast infections from your life. I must warn you that this is not an overnight fix. It will require some effort on your part. The system that I will describe was developed through many years of study and research and has been proven by thousands of yeast infection sufferers...including myself.

We will now focus on eliminating the root cause of your yeast problems. We are going to change the environment within your body so that yeast infections can no longer thrive. We are also going to discuss changes in the external environment in ways that will strengthen you against any future yeast overgrowth.

As we have discussed earlier, yeast is a living, growing organism. It exists in our bodies for a purpose and as long as it is kept under control it is harmless. The natural processes within our bodies are usually able to keep the yeast under control. The only way to permanently eliminate yeast infections is to be sure that we never provide an environment within our bodies that allows the yeast to thrive and grow out of control.

This will be a 100% natural process and I have tried very hard to only recommend products that are commonly available, either in your home or at local stores. A few of the items can be ordered online and I have tried to provide good reliable sources for those. I recommend no over-the-counter or prescription medications and I have kept the cost as low as possible.

My guarantee to you is that if you follow the steps as they are presented you will feel healthier, younger, more energized, and better all over. I know it works because it is basically the same process I followed to become yeast free and I have helped many other women and men to follow. I have seen the positive results time and time again.

Natural, holistic healing requires thinking about all the parts of your life system - physical, mental, and emotional, because these are connected and all affect your overall health and your body's ability to respond to and defeat infections. Instead of concentrating on each part separately we will treat them as a whole. By treating yeast infections holistically we will replace the bad bacteria with natural helper bacteria so that your body regains a healthy balance of the bacterial count.

Holistic healing also focuses on all the things around you, including your environment and the people you interact with. For example, if you have a vaginal infection it is important to treat your partner – especially in cases of chronic yeast infections. Having your doctor say to you, "Here is your pill, see you later," will not cure the yeast infection. Yeast infections are easily passed back and forth between partners and in many cases, especially in men, the infection does not cause symptoms. Treating your partner, using condoms, and avoiding tight fitting clothing are all examples of a holistic approach to treatment.

We will learn to recognize and control anything -- poor diet, drugs, alcohol, stress, fatigue -- which lowers your body's natural resistance to disease.

There are 4 steps to the Yeast Free Life plan and we will discuss each of them in detail.

Step 1 (Diet and Supplementation) and Step 2 (Killing Existing Candida) should be started at the same time.

Step 2 will be completed in 3 weeks, after which you will begin Step 3 (Internal Cleansing)

Step 4 (Adding Friendly Bacteria) will start after Step 3 is completed.

It is important to understand that all four steps must be performed in this order to ensure that your yeast infections will never return. We will follow a logical process that starts with diet/supplementation and eliminating any Candida overgrowth that is in your body. The point of this step is to beat back any overgrowth that may have already taken place and weaken the Candida so we can easily defeat it by changing the body's internal environment and cleansing it to make it more able to fight off future Candida attacks. The 4 steps are:

Step 1 - Diet and Supplementation

    What you should not eat.

    What you should eat.

    What supplements you should take.

Step 2 - Kill any existing Candida overgrowth

Step 3 - Internal Cleansing

    Colon Cleansing

    Parasite Cleansing

    Liver/Gall Bladder Flush

Step 4 - Adding Friendly Bacteria

Now, let's get started...

STEP 1 – Diet and Supplementation
(START STEPS 1 and 2 AT THE SAME TIME)

Diet

One of the most important steps we can take in changing our internal environment and achieving the Yeast Free Life is to change what we put into our bodies through our diet. While you don't have to completely change the way you eat forever it is necessary to give up some things for awhile and, yes, some things forever. Some of these may be your favorite things so this might be the hardest step you have to take to be completely yeast free. You will probably be amazed, however, at how fast your yeast symptoms (and many other health-related symptoms) will change just by making simple dietary changes.

We will address diet from 2 different directions... (1) what you should not eat and; (2) what you should eat.

What You <u>Should Not</u> Eat

White Sugar - You must eliminate refined (white) sugar from your diet. Yeast loves white sugar. You probably love it too. "Friendly" bacteria, your immune system, and your organs do not love white sugar. When sugar cane is processed to make white sugar it is stripped of its fiber and nutrients. White sugar is a chemical element that is simply not even recognized by our bodies. It robs the body of vitamins and minerals and causes blood sugar levels to spike. Sugar causes the pancreas to produce excess amounts of insulin which, in turn, results in low blood sugar levels, low energy, and fatigue.

When sugar is eaten the body produces extra hormones to metabolize the glucose. These extra hormones stress the liver and create a hormonal imbalance in the body. The liver also converts the sugar into long-chain fats that pollute the blood. These two conditions help to create an environment in which Candida can rapidly grow and flourish.

Sugar also has a damaging effect on the immune system which severely affects the body's ability to defend itself against bad bacteria and the overgrowth of Candida. It stresses the liver, often causing it to enlarge, and creates an acidic environment in the stomach...all of which contribute to Candida growth and yeast infections.

Refined Carbohydrates - Avoid white flour, white rice, white pasta, and all refined, puffed, or extruded grains or cereals. The sugars in refined carbohydrates are fast acting and can cause the same effects as eating plain white sugar. These refined foods have had their nutritious vitamin and mineral filled pulp removed leaving only a glue-like substance that clogs the digestive tract, pollutes the blood, and contributes to Candida growth.

Substitute brown rice, whole rye, and other whole, refined grains and you will notice a decrease in yeast infection symptoms and better overall health.

Bakers Yeast and Fermented Foods - Avoid bread, pizza, cakes, vinegar, and all malted products. This includes pastries, buns, rolls, biscuits, crackers, soy sauce, mushrooms, stuffing mixes and anything breaded. Don't eat any nutritional supplement not labeled as yeast-free. Avoid miso, tempeh, nuts not in their shell (avoid peanuts altogether), smoked and processed meats, and foods containing MSG (mono sodium glutamate). Notice that I said "avoid" not "eliminate." It is not necessary for you to completely eliminate all of these items from your diet. It is important, though, to be aware that these items often contain yeast or fungus, which is exactly what we are trying to get rid of.

These items also frequently contain hydrogenated oil which can clog the liver, spleen, muscles, and kidneys and create fatty deposits and dangerous toxic buildup.

Dairy Products - Eliminate anything made from cow's milk. Dairy products are one of the worst yeast infection-aggravating products. Milk products cause allergies, heavy mucus, and digestive tract clogging. Maybe more importantly, all commercial dairy cattle are injected with hormones and antibiotics to increase their milk yield. Some of these hormones and antibiotics are passed into the milk. When we consume dairy products we are introducing these toxic products into our own bodies.

Also, pasteurized milk contains beta lactose, which is quickly absorbed into the blood and has an effect on the body almost identical to that experience when refined sugar is eaten.

You should avoid milk, cheese, and products that contain lactose, milk proteins, whey protein, and dry skim milk powder. Goat's and sheep's milk are acceptable alternatives to cow's milk. Sesame seed butter, soy products, and nut milks are also good substitutes.

Alcohol - All alcohol weakens the immune system. Beer is especially bad because it is made primarily with yeast and grains. Wine is also fermented using yeast and it may also be high in sugar. Alcohol will slow or damage liver function and slow metabolism, creating an environment in which Candida can expand.

Nicotine and Other Stimulants - Tobacco contains fungal residues and it also robs the body of the oxygen that cells require to fight infection. Coffee and tea have a negative effect on your adrenal glands and can create a hormonal imbalance. They put a strain on your immune system during a time when you want to give it all the support you can. Green or herbal tea is a good substitute for caffeinated coffee or tea.

What You <u>Should</u> Eat

Non-animal Protein - It is best to cut out animal meat entirely if you can but if you must eat it, it is best to buy organic meat. Make sure it is labeled organic. If it isn't, it is not organic. Non-organic meat is highly contaminated with residues of hormones and antibiotics. Of non-organically raised meat, wild game and lamb are the safest. Chicken is the most contaminated meat. Tasty meat alternatives exist, including TVP (textured vegetable protein) and soy-based "meat" products.

Fruits – Fruits that do not have a high sugar level can be eaten in moderation. Eat the fruit raw and, where possible, with the skin. Some good, nutritious, blood-cleansing fruits are apples, grapes, grapefruits, lemons, limes, peaches/pears, strawberries, tangerines, avocadoes, blackberries, blueberries, and watermelon. Fruits should always be eaten raw and fresh…never frozen, canned, dried, or cooked. All fruit has some sugar content so servings should be limited to 1 per day. If you have severe yeast infection or are having problems eliminating the yeast infection symptoms it is best to eliminate fruit from your diet completely.

Nuts - Almonds, Brazil nuts, Macadamia nuts, pecans, and walnuts are just fine. Completely avoid peanuts, peanut butter, and anything made with peanuts or peanut oil.

Whole Grains – Whole grains are complex carbohydrates and great sources of protein. Whole grains are not only low in fat; they are high in fiber, vitamins, and minerals. Healthy whole grains include millet, brown rice, quinoa (pronounced "keenwa"), barley, rye, and buckwheat.

Fresh, Organic Vegetables - Raw or steamed vegetables are the best. You can consume unlimited amounts of non-starchy vegetables such as peppers, cucumbers, lettuce, celery, cauliflower, broccoli, cabbage, spinach, and Brussels sprouts. The complex carbohydrates in these vegetables help regulate your blood sugar levels and provide a steady source of energy.

Beans - Beans are a good source of protein. If they are difficult to digest, soak them in water for a day or two and cook them slowly over low heat. Try lentils or green split peas. If you buy canned beans make sure there is no added sugar.

Fish – Fish is an excellent substitute for red meat. Cold water fish such as tuna and salmon are high in protein and are a good source of essential fatty acids.

Cold-pressed Oils - If you can cook with or include these oils as ingredients for your meals, you can count on their antifungal powers in the diet. These include flaxseed oil, olive oil, sesame oil, and sunflower oil. Remember that peanut oil, or any blend that includes peanut oil, is not allowed.

Water - Drink lots of water every day. Drinking at least 2 liters of water each day is necessary for cleansing and detoxifying. Fresh water will flush the toxins from the primary organs and prevent toxic buildup which leads to Candida overgrowth. Drinking substantial quantities of water will also keep the kidneys clean and help discharge waste and prevent kidney stones.

Garlic - Garlic is an antifungal and a decongestant. It also helps increase our vitamin absorption and helps eliminate toxins from our body. Garlic is a perfect anti-yeast medicine. Try to eat it raw. If you can't stand the taste, use small cloves or cut smaller pieces and swallow them whole. Don't use odorless or heat treated garlic. The active ingredient, allicin gives garlic its odor. Allicin is destroyed by heat.

Garlic has anti-microbial powers against various types of bacteria and fungi. The insulin found in garlic is a type of fiber that the friendly intestinal bacterium loves. Garlic has powerful medicinal effects and its antiseptic properties can help purify the blood.

The Die-Off Process (Herx Reaction)

The purpose of these diet changes is to begin to starve the Candida that remains in your system. This "starving" causes them to die out. This process is known as "die off." Unfortunately, die off often means that your symptoms will seem to temporarily get worse.

When you start the process of starving Candida, the yeast will do everything it can to try to survive. After all, it is a living organism that has had control of your body for a long time. It will fight to preserve itself and to keep from being killed. The worst thing you can do is quit your diet and supplements during this time! Even if the feeling is unpleasant, you'll know your actions are starting to take effect.

While some people experience little or no symptoms during the die off process others report flu-like symptoms. Some of these symptoms might include:

- Nausea
- Irritability
- Headaches
- Gas
- Loss of energy

- Craving sugar
- Blurred vision

You are experiencing what health care professionals call the Herx reaction. The Jarisch-Herxheimer reaction (Herx) is your body's response to the dying off of yeast and bacteria. It means you're getting better. The dying organisms are releasing toxins into your body faster than your body can get rid of them. The wastes and poisons from the dying colonies may have been in your body for years. This process happens naturally as your body begins to heal itself.

In order to minimize the effects of the Herx reaction, make sure you are getting at least 1.5 liters of water a day, eating plenty of fresh vegetables, consuming 1 tbsp of ground flaxseed per day to keep the intestines moving and getting exercise daily. Stretching exercises such as yoga can be especially beneficial.

Because these symptoms may be similar to the ones you are experiencing from your yeast infections, it may seem like the disease is getting worse instead of better. But this is actually a good sign. These symptoms may last a few days, or even a few weeks, depending on how much the Candida has spread throughout your system. You can rest assured, however, that they are only temporary and the last, dieing fight from the Candida that you will be free of for the rest of your life.

Supplements

It would be great if we could be assured of getting all the vitamins and minerals that we need to fight yeast infections from our daily diet. Unfortunately, due to the way that foods are grown, preserved, processed, and prepared it is nearly impossible to get the vitamins and minerals our body needs from the foods we eat.

Now that we have altered our diet to eliminate the yeast-causing foods and added the yeast-fighting foods it is time to compliment our body with essential vitamins, minerals, and special supplements to boost our immune system and to give it the energy it needs to get rid of toxins and fight Candida.

I suggest you take the following supplements on a daily basis. These supplements will significantly improve your yeast infection symptoms, boost your mental abilities, increase your energy and vibrancy, and improve your emotional outlook.

1. Essential Fatty Acid (EFAs)

EFAs are an important supplement to a healthy Candida-fighting diet. They are rich in omega-3, omega-6, and omega-9 compounds, which have rich antifungal properties. EFAs are found in flax oil, cold water fish such as salmon or tuna, sunflower seeds, soybean, borage, walnut, and safflower oil. Recent research suggests that ingredients in EFAs are also effective for treatment of immune system diseases such as lupus and other autoimmune diseases.

There are a couple of reasons that essential fatty acids are used in the treatment of yeast infections. First, they act as antifungal agents in the body, which combats the growth of yeast. Secondly, EFA oils such as flaxseed oil are helpful in the repair of Leaky Gut Syndrome. Tests have shown that the ingestion of these oils makes the intestine less porous, which stops those undigested bits of food from passing through the intestine and prohibits these toxins from entering the bloodstream. This can begin the healing of your digestive tract from the damage caused by the rhizoids ("legs") in the fungal form of Candida.

Even a healthy western diet is almost always deficient in omega-3. Omega-3 EFAs can be obtained by eating walnuts, cod liver oil, and salmon. However, because of high mercury levels in fish there is a limit of how much we should eat. The only way to be sure we are getting enough EFA's, especially omega-3, is to use a supplement.

I recommend a product called "Complete Essential Fatty Acids" which is available at:

http://NaturalLifeSuperstore.com/efa.html

Take 1 softgel capsule 3 times per day tablespoons per day.

2. B-Complex Vitamins

The B-Complex vitamins, B-1 (thiamin, B-2 (riboflavin), B-3 (niacin), B-5 (pantothenic acid, and B-6 (pyridoxine) are essential in controlling yeast infections. These vitamins are responsible for healthy nerves, skin, and eyes and for metabolizing and digesting food.

I recommend using "B-Complex Sustained Release" which you can order from:

http://NaturalLifeSuperstore.com/b-complex.html

3. Vitamin C

Vitamin C is a powerful antioxidant that protects essential fatty acids. It is effective in neutralizing toxins and reducing stress and speeds healing of damaged tissue. Vitamin C is naturally found in red bell peppers, oranges, lemons, watermelons, kiwi, strawberries, green leafy vegetables, broccoli, and parsley.
I RECOMMEND USING 1500 mg per day of a timed-released product such as the one available here:

http://NaturalLifeSuperstore.com/vitamin-c.html

4. Colostrum

Colostrum is rich in immunoglobulin, which provides essential growth and immune factors that aid overall health. It is one of the most effective supplements to support the immune system. Research has shown that Colostrum has powerful natural immune and growth factors that bring the body to a state of homeostasis, its powerful, vital natural state of health and well being. Colostrum helps support healthy immune function; it also enables us to resist the harmful effects of pollutants, contaminants and allergens where they attack us. Plus, the growth factors in Colostrum create an enhanced ability to metabolize or "burn" fat, greater ease in building lean muscle mass, and enhanced rejuvenation of skin and muscle.

I recommend Bovine Colostrum which is nearly identical to human colostrum but is 4 times richer in immune factors. Bovine Colostrum can be purchased at:

http://NaturalLifeSuperstore.com/colostrum.html

5. Coconut Oil

Coconut oil is extremely beneficial in controlling Candida. Since the 1960s, coconut oil has been mistakenly described as unhealthy. The media reported on studies finding that tropical coconut oils were laden with artery-clogging fats. What went unreported was the fact that the coconut oil used in the studies was hydrogenated—not the virgin oil used for centuries as a staple food. Coconut oil is about 50 percent lauric acid, a rare medium-chain fatty acid found in mother's milk that supports healthy metabolism and is now being studied for its anti-fungal, anti-viral, and anti-bacterial health-protecting properties.

I recommend adding 1 or 2 tablespoons per day of Organic Virgin Coconut Oil to your food. You can purchase coconut oil at health stores (be sure you are getting "organic virgin" coconut oil) or order from:

http://NaturalLifeSuperstore.com/coconutoil.html

6. Blue-Green Algae

Blue-Green Algae is naturally rich in amino acids, minerals, vitamins, fatty acids, chlorophyll and protein and may help increase energy, decrease fatigue, enhance brain function, oxygenate the blood, nourish the nervous system, improve memory and concentration, increase muscle mass, speed healing, protect against pollutants and radiation, purify the blood, prevent kidney stones, and improve over-all health.

This supplement will significantly improve your digestive systems and help remove heavy metals from your body. It increases the alkalinity of the digestive systems, boosts friendly bacteria, and helps with cleansing the bowels.

I recommend using a concentrated blue-green algae product called Spirulina which is available at health stores and at:

http://NaturalLifeSuperstore.com/spirulina.html

STEP 2 – Kill Existing Candida Overgrowth

As you begin to adjust your diet and add the vitamins and supplements your body needs to resist future yeast infections it is important to, once-and-for-all, get rid of any remaining Candida overgrowth that is in your body. It is very important to do this so that you don't allow any remaining yeast cells to reset themselves and begin to grow again.

While there are antifungal products that will kill existing Candida, the safest and most effective way to do the job is by using fiber digesting enzymes to attack the Candida cell walls.

I highly recommend a product called Candida Clear because it is extremely effective and has no negative side effects. Candida Clear contains no anti-fungal drugs, so it cannot damage the liver as anti-fungal drugs often do. It does not cause the yeast to react chemically, so that die off reactions do not occur. Because it digests the yeast's cell wall, and because the yeast cannot change its basic cellular structure, the yeast develops no resistance to it. It provides only cellulast enzymes, so that it's completely safe. It controls localized yeast infections within three days. It provides profound improvement against deep, systemic problems within 6 to 30 days.

Because the cell wall of Candida (and all other fungal organisms) is made mostly of fiber, fiber digesting enzymes can break it down. As this occurs, the yeast dies. While Candida and other yeasts can develop immunity to anti-fungal drugs and herbs, it has no defense against enzymes. Thus, enzymes are the best possible solution.

Candida Clear has a blend of plant based, fiber digesting enzymes that attack and destroy the cell wall of the Candida cells. The important thing to know is that, since Candida Clear is not an anti-fungal there is no die off effect that is sometimes experienced with other treatments.

Candida Clear is taken as directed on the package at a rate of 2 capsules per day for 2 weeks.

Candida Clear is available in some health stores and several online sites including:

http://NaturalLifeSuperstore.com/candida.html

STEP 3 – Internal Cleansing

We have taken the steps necessary to kill the remaining Candida overgrowth and we have adjusted your diet to be sure you are not creating a good environment for yeast to grow in the future. It is now time to lay the foundation for your Yeast Free Life by cleansing and regenerating your important internal organs.

A good cleansing program will not only eliminate yeast infections. It will also eliminate many other disease symptoms including chronic pain, hair loss, and skin disorders. It will boost your mental clarity and get rid of that "foggy mind" that so many people suffer from. Finally, it will give you an amazing boost of energy and possibly change your entire outlook on life.

When the digestive system becomes sluggish and over-toxic it becomes weak and inefficient. Toxic bowels lead to blood intoxication and a sluggish liver. A weak and sluggish liver is incapable of handling the over-acidity and toxic overload will release toxins to other parts of the body such as the kidneys, heart, brain, skin, and lymph. This results in disease symptoms related to the organ where toxins have settled. Before any disease such as yeast infection can be permanently defeated, these toxins must be removed.

A deep cleansing program will help the body release toxins from the liver, kidneys, and gallbladder, and the blood and lymph systems. The liver cleanse will strengthen and boost the function of these vital organs of elimination, resulting in a more balanced and effective internal system capable of self-healing and handling many conditions, including yeast infections.

We will follow a 3 step process for complete inner body cleansing. It is very important that the cleanses be performed in the order listed.

1. Colon Cleansing

A good cleansing program should always begin by removing the waste in your colon, the last portion of your food processing chain. If you attempt to clean your liver, blood, or lymph system without first addressing a waste filled bowel, the excreted toxins will only get recycled back into your body.

One of the most frequent bowel problems that people experience today is constipation. Constipation is generally attributed to a low fiber diet and lack of sufficient water, which cause our fecal matter to become condensed and compressed.

A constipated system is one in which the transition, or "time", of toxic wastes is slow and the consistency of the stool can cause strain (which over time may cause hemorrhoids, varicose veins, hernia, or other mechanically induced problems). The longer the "transit time", the longer the toxic waste matter sits in our bowel which allows proteins to putrefy, fats to become rancid, and carbohydrates to ferment.

The longer your body is exposed to putrefying food in your intestines, the greater the risk of developing disease. Even with one bowel movement per day, you will still have at least three meals worth of waste matter putrefying in your colon at all times. On top of all this, your system can also become continuously self-polluting by the poisonous gases that are caused by foods you don't tolerate. These poisonous gases can enter your bloodstream, irritating your organs and joints.

Alternating between constipation and diarrhea, or diarrhea alone, are also indications of foul matter in your intestines. And finally, the much more serious problems of cancer and immune system dysfunctions begin with a toxic bowel.

The long held belief of some health professionals is that many people just have fewer bowel movements than others. This is true, but they also neglected to inform these individuals that those having fewer bowel movements are harboring a fertile breeding ground for serious diseases and possibly death. Infrequent or poor quality bowel movements over an extended period of time are very hazardous to your health.

Colon cleansing can be accomplished in one of two ways...by using an enema or by taking a natural herbal colon cleansing product by mouth. The two methods are equally effective. Some people prefer the enema because it is faster and a little less expensive while others do not like the slight discomfort and inconvenience involved in using an enema. Personally, I prefer to use a natural herbal product.

The method you use to cleanse your colon really is a matter of personal preference. How you accomplish the cleansing is not nearly as important as that you DO IT! Unless you eliminate the waste in your colon it will be reabsorbed into your system and retoxify your blood and organs.

Natural Herbal Colon Cleansing - If you decide to use a natural herbal product I recommend a product the 7 Day Colon Cleanse. The 7 Day Colon Cleanse Kit includes 21 packets of capsules. You simply take one packet 3 times per day for 7 days. You can buy the 7 Day Colon Cleanse Kit at:

http://NaturalLifeSuperstore.com/colon-cleanse.html

Remember to drink plenty of water!

Enema Colon Cleansing - As an alternative to using a natural herbal product you can rinse your colon with water by using an enema. Enemas are cheap and can easily be done in the comfort and privacy of your home. An enema works simply by rinsing your colon with water. I recommend using a water bag enema. Here is the process for doing it:

> 1. Rinse the enema bag and fill it with warm (not cold and not hot) water to which you have added 1 teaspoon of salt and 1 teaspoon of baking soda.
>
> 2. Perform the enema in each of 3 positions...(a) lying on your left side with knees drawn toward your chest, (b) lying on your right side with knees drawn toward your chest, and (c) kneeling with your forehead on the floor and your buttocks up. Doing the enema in these 3 positions will ensure that you are covering the entire colon.
>
> 3. Use a lubricant gel such as Vaseline to lubricate the enema tip and fully insert it into the anus. Slowly and gently empty about half of the enema bag into your colon. This should not be painful but it is normal to experience slight cramps. If it is painful or very uncomfortable, you should stop the process and relax a little before continuing. Hold the water in for 3 to 5 minutes or until you feel an urgent need to expel it.
>
> 4. Repeat the process for the other 2 positions.

2. Parasite Cleansing

No cleansing protocol is complete until you kill the parasites that inhabit your system. Parasites are living organisms that live within your body. They eat, lay eggs, and secrete toxins into your bloodstream. They live off of your body and the food you supply them and can grow and multiply continuously without you ever knowing it.

As the parasites grow and reproduce inside your body they steel vital nutrients and minerals that you need to be healthy. They eat essential protein and damage your lungs, joints, nervous system, and liver.

The most effective and natural way to get rid of these nasty parasites is by taking a combination of wormwood, cloves, black walnut, and garlic. If you do this you will kill most or all of the parasites living within your body.

There are numerous products available at health stores and pharmacies to help in your parasite cleansing. The best product I have found is called Parasite Complex. It is widely available in some stores and online and can be ordered at this site:

http://NaturalLifeSuperstore.com/parasite-cleanse.html

3. Liver/Gallbladder Flush

The liver is an important detoxifier and must be thoroughly cleansed. The bile, which is stored in the gallbladder in a concentrated form, is of extreme importance in all areas of the body. The gallbladder actually draws the bile into itself from the liver duct. Many physical problems are the direct result of inadequate bile flow. The synovial fluid around all joints will decrease if bile flow is low, sometimes causing terrible pain. Many people will take cortisone injections for relief believing it, mistakenly, to be arthritis or some other inflammatory disease. The cure of course comes with liver cleansing.

Another area of the body that can suffer from lack of bile is the sinuses. This soothing lubricant (bile) keeps mucus membranes from becoming dry and inflamed. Most allergy conditions can be traced to liver congestion. Avoiding foods that create a reaction bring relief, but will not cure the allergy. Allergies and sinus conditions will often disappear after the liver has been cleansed.

Also, the body begins to suffer the effects of poor assimilation of fat-soluble nutrients, which may play a role in the development of yeast infections, eczema, psoriasis, dry skin, falling hair, tendonitis, night blindness, accumulations of calcium in tissues, and sometimes prostate enlargement in men. Hemorrhoids due to blockage of the portal vein draining the liver are often the result of this congestion.

The importance of cleansing debris from the liver and the gall bladder, thus keeping the bile free flowing, cannot be overemphasized. This can be accomplished by doing the Liver - Gall Bladder Flush. There are four basic ingredients in this procedure.

Ingredients You Will Need:

A. Apple juice, which acts as a solvent in the bile to weaken adhesions between solid globules. The apple juice should be natural, unfiltered, and free of additives and preservatives.

B. 4 tablespoons Epsom salts (Magnesium sulfate), allows magnesium to be absorbed into the bloodstream, relaxing smooth muscles. Large solid particles which otherwise might create spasms are able to pass through a relaxed bile duct.

C. 1/2 Cup Extra Virgin Olive Oil, which stimulates the gall bladder and bile duct to contract powerfully, thus expelling solid particles that may have been kept in storage for years.

D. 1 large or 2 small grapefruits or 3 lemons, the acidic juice speeds the transit of the olive oil thru the stomach and into the duodenum, which helps prevent or minimize nausea.

The Process:

The steps in doing this are not difficult and are as follows:

1. For 5 days prior to the "Flush" consume as much apple juice or cider as the appetite permits, in addition to regular meals. Nutritional supplements should also be taken during this time. For the last two days (day 4 and 5) try to take 8 ounces of apple juice every two hours until at least 1/2 gallon each day has been taken.

2. On the sixth day... Eat a no-fat breakfast and lunch such as cooked cereal with fruit, fruit juice, bread, and (no butter or milk), baked potato, or other vegetables with sea salt only. This allows the bile to build up and develop pressure in the liver. Higher pressure pushes out more stones.

2:00 PM
Get your Epsom salts ready. Mix 4 tbsp. in 3 cups water and pour this into a jar. Do not eat or drink after 2 o'clock. If you break this rule you could feel quite ill.

6:00 PM
Drink one serving (3/4 cup) of the cold Epsom salts. If you did not prepare this ahead of time, do it right now. You may also add 1/8 tbsp. vitamin C powdered to improve the taste. You may also drink a few mouthfuls of water afterwards or rinse your mouth. Get the olive oil and grapefruit out of the refrigerator to warm up.

8:00 PM
Repeat by drinking another 3/4 cup of Epsom salts. You haven't eaten since two o'clock, but you won't feel hungry. Get your bedtime chores done. The timing is critical for success; don't be more than 10 minutes early or late.

9:45 PM
Pour 1/2 cup (measured) olive oil into a pint jar. Squeeze the grapefruit by hand into the measuring cup. Remove pulp

with fork. You should have at least 1/2 cup, but up to 3/4 cup is best. Add this to the olive oil. Close the jar tightly with the lid and shake hard until watery (only fresh grapefruit does this).

10:00 PM
Drink the potion you have mixed. Drinking through a large plastic straw helps it go down easier. Take it to your bedside if you want, but drink it standing up. Get it down within 5 minutes (fifteen minutes for very elderly or weak persons).

Lie down immediately!!! You might fail to get stones out if you don't. The sooner you lie down the more stones you will get out. Be ready for bed ahead of time. Don't clean up the kitchen. As soon as the drink is down walk to your bed and lie on the right side with the right knee drawn up toward the chin for at least 20 minutes (you can briefly stretch your right leg, if necessary) or lie down flat on your back with your head up high on the pillow for 20 minutes before going to sleep. This encourages the oil to drain from the stomach, helping contents of the gall bladder and/or liver to move into the small intestine. Try to think about what is happening in the liver. Try to keep perfectly still for at least 20 minutes.

You may feel a train of stones traveling along the bile ducts like marbles. There is no pain because the bile duct valves are open (thank you Epsom salts!). Go to sleep. You may fail to get stones out if you don't.

Next Morning
Upon awakening take your third 3/4 cup dose of Epsom salts. If you have indigestion or nausea wait unit it is gone before drinking the Epsom salts. You may go back to bed. Don't take this potion before 6:00 AM.

2 Hours Later
Take your fourth (the last) dose of Epsom salts. Drink 3/4 cup of the mixture. You may go back to bed.

After 2 More Hours You May Eat
Start with fresh fruit juice. Half an hour later eat fruit. One hour later you may eat regular food, but keep it light. By supper you should feel recovered.

How well did you do?

Expect diarrhea in the morning. Use a flashlight to look for gallstones in the toilet with the bowel movement. Look for the green kind since this is proof that they are genuine gallstones, not food residue. Only bile from the liver is pea green. The bowel movement sinks, but gallstones float because of the cholesterol inside. The first cleanse may rid you of them for a few days, but as the stones from the rear travel forward, they give you the same symptoms again. You may repeat cleanses at two week intervals.

Note: If one should vomit during the consumption of the oil and juice, the procedure should be continued until it is finished. It is not necessary to make up for the amount that was vomited. Nausea felt during this process usually indicates stimulation of the gall bladder and/or liver.

You should not be frightened by the above references to nausea, vomiting, soreness of abdomen, etc.

Chances are that the symptoms won't be severe enough to cause vomiting or soreness of the abdomen, as this happens only very rarely. Many people complete this procedure with minimal discomfort, and nearly everyone feels better after completing it.

Often times, persons suffering for years from gallstones, lack of appetite, biliousness, backaches, nausea, and a host of other complaints will find gallstones-type objects in the stool the day following the flush.

These objects are light to dark green in color, very irregular in shape, gelatinous in texture, and of sizes varying from "grape seed size" to "cherry size". When a large volume of gall stones is seen, the liver flush should be repeated in 2 weeks.

Generally, the liver flush is repeated at 2 - 4 week intervals until the volume of gall stones seen (each time) has been greatly reduced. This can require 10 - 15 flushes, or more, because your liver will be "pulling" cholesterol out of your body, where it may have accumulated for many years or decades. After the initial series, repeat the liver flush 2 times per year, for "maintenance."

STEP 4 – Adding Friendly Bacteria

If you have followed the first 3 steps you have now killed your Candida, changed your diet, and cleansed your bowels and internal organs. You should now be Candida free and well on the path to a Yeast Free Life. Now we are ready to flood your system with good, friendly bacteria.

It is important that we reintroduce good bacteria or "probiotics" into your body to reestablish a balanced bacterial environment in your intestine. Keeping the bacteria in balance will prevent any resurfacing of Candida.

Probiotics

Probiotics are strains of live bacteria that will help you to regain those "good" bacteria that prevent the overgrowth of yeast. It is important for the body to contain "good" bacteria to ensure the best condition of the intestinal tract and the immune system.

It is important to make sure your bowels are well populated with probiotics so that they are prepared to kill parasites and

Candida. Establishing and maintaining a good probiotic population in the bowels is absolutely essential in ensuring that a Candida overgrowth is never again allowed to occur.

On a daily basis, the human body has to protect itself from invasion of undesirable organisms and thus it is critical to maintain a proper balance of micro flora throughout the bacterial ecosystem of the intestinal tract. Keeping an ample population of beneficial bacteria (probiotics) throughout the intestinal tract will help to protect intestinal integrity and thus strengthen overall health.

Daily consumption of probiotic foods and probiotic supplements will ensure that you are ingesting proper amounts of "friendly" bacteria.

Probiotic microorganisms are cultured in a laboratory and shipped alive in some yogurts and supplements. The microorganisms are able to stay alive as they pass through your system and they live in your intestines. Having these probiotics in your systems supports good digestion, enhances the immune system, increases resistance to infection, and fights off bad bacteria and fungus (including Candida).

There are 2 primary ways to get probiotics into your body. One is by eating **yogurt** (but not just any yogurt) and the other is through **supplements**.

Yogurt – Much has been written and advertised about the advantages of eating yogurt to establish a good probiotic balance…and some of it is true. The problem with most yogurts sold in stores is that it does not have any living probiotics. While all yogurt starts off having probiotics, the vast amount of mass produced yogurt is heated in production. While this heating does extend the shelf life of the yogurt it also kills all the friendly bacteria. Although the labels on most commercial yogurt will say that it is "made with active cultures" (which it is) the label will not say that most or all of the active cultures are dead. Dead cultures do nothing to help the probiotic balance.

Be sure your yogurt package says that it contains "live and active cultures." This indicates a live starter culture was used. For the added benefit of probiotics, look for LACTOBACILLUS ACIDOPHILUS, L. CASEI, L. REUTERI or BIFIDOBACTERIUM BIFIDUM on the ingredients list. L. acidophilus is by far the most commonly added probiotic, featured in such favorites as Dannon, Columbo, Yoplait, and Breyers.

The problem with these products...and the reason I really do not recommend yogurt as your main probiotic source. is that they are typically overly laden with sugar. If you are going to use yogurt as you source for probiotics please use only yogurt that is not heated and contains no sugar, additives, or coloring.

Supplements -

Option 1 – Primal Defense Ultra

Primal Defense Ultra is a whole food probiotic blend containing 14 strains of plant based, non-dairy Homeostatic Soil Organisms (HSOs). HSOs contain naturally occurring live enzymes, vitamins and minerals designed to optimize the digestive terrain, bowel and immune system function. These micro-organisms will eliminate undigested matter, yeast, parasites and bad bacteria from the intestines. Primal Defense contains the same nutrients used for thousands of years by some of the healthiest and longest living people in the world.
Beneficial soil and plant based microbes used to be ingested through food grown

in rich, unpolluted soil. However, for the last 50 years our soil has been sterilized with pesticides and herbicides, destroying most bacteria, both bad and good. Our modern lifestyle, which includes antibiotics, chlorinated water, agricultural chemicals, pollution, and poor diet, is responsible for eradicating much of the beneficial bacteria in our bodies. A lack of beneficial microorganisms often results in poor intestinal and immune system health, contributing to a wide range of symptoms and illnesses.

Adults should take 1 caplet three times per day with 8 oz of water. It works best when taken on an empty stomach.

Primal Defense Ultra can be purchased at some pharmacies and health stores and at many online sites including:

http://NaturalLifeSuperstore.com/primal.html

Option 2 – Suprema Dophilus Multi Probiotic

Another excellent alternative is Suprema Dophilus Multi Probiotic which contains 8 different viable bacterial strains totaling 4 billion good viable bacteria per capsule. Suprema Dophilus Multi Probiotic contains several forma of Acidophilus (Lactobacillus acidophilus) which is a

friendly intestinal flora that promotes intestinal health, assists in the digestion of proteins, has anti-fungal activity, and helps with Candida overgrowth, yeast infections, urinary tract infections, cholesterol levels, lactose intolerance, nutrient assimilation, detoxification, post-antibiotic treatment, constipation and diarrhea control, bad breath, gas, and intestinal disorders.
Supreme Dophilus Multi Probiotic can be purchased at some pharmacies and health stores and some online sites including:

http://NaturalLifeSuperstore.com/acidophilus.html

7. A FINAL WORD

Thank you for sticking with me through this book. I hope you have a much better understanding of what yeast infection is, what causes it, and how to eliminate it from your life. I also hope that you have tried some of the 12 hour relief methods to get rid of your immediate symptoms. Most of all, I hope you have committed to doing what is necessary to permanently eliminate yeast infections and that you are on your way to a Yeast Free Life.

It should be clear by now that, although yeast infections cause external symptoms, they are really a result of internal problems. The symptoms we feel from yeast infections are, in fact, warning signs from our body that we have a potentially serious internal imbalance.

Using creams, lotions, or medications to treat the symptoms may help to reduce the symptoms in the short-run but will not lead to a permanent solution. Only when we tackle the problem from the inside will we ever be able to cure the root cause of the problem.

If you seriously adopt the necessary dietary changes, supplementation, cleansing, and life-style changes you will fix the internal problem that is causing your yeast infections. To treat the infections in any other way is simply to mask the symptoms and risk even worse problems in the future.

Achieving a well-balanced system isn't easy and it will take some effort and sacrifice. The benefit, however, is a healthy body and a more vibrant, energetic, stronger, and happier life.

The solution is now in your hands. I very much appreciate the time you have spent reading my book. I wish you happiness, success, blessings, and, of course, a Yeast Free Life.

Sarah

Appendix 1 - CONVENTIONAL DRUGS AND TREATMENTS

Introduction

Hardly a day goes by that I do not receive an email asking for my opinion about one of the many yeast infection drugs that are on the market. My answer usually includes the following advice:

1. Drugs, both over-the-counter and prescription, are rarely needed to cure yeast infections.

2. Drugs may give temporary relief but, because they treat the symptoms and not the root cause, they are not a permanent cure.

3. Drugs often do more harm than good.

4. Consult your doctor about the drugs you are taking or considering taking.

5. ALL DRUGS HAVE NEGATIVE SIDE EFFECTS. DO NOT TAKE A DRUG IF YOU DO NOT UNDERSTAND THESE SIDE EFFECTS.

Item number 5 concerns me greatly. I think that far too many people assume a drug is safe because the doctor prescribes it or because an actor on television tells us it is okay to use.

Through my research I discovered that every single drug used to treat yeast infections is dangerous. Each and every one of these drugs can cause serious health issues or even death.

If you ever consider using any of these drugs it is absolutely necessary that you understand the potential side effects, possible drug interactions, and the risks involved. Only after understanding the possible effects should you use any of these drugs.

On the following pages I have listed the potential side effects and other warnings associated with the most popular drugs used to treat yeast infections. I have provided this information for your information and as an aid in your decision making. As always, please consult your doctor if you have any questions about your medical treatment.

Amphocin

Amphocin can have serious side effects and should only be used for treatment of patients with progressive and potentially life-threatening fungal infections. It should not be used to treat noninvasive forms of fungal disease such as oral thrush, vaginal yeast infections and esophageal yeast infections.

Amphocin is a brand name for the drug Amphotericin B.

Use of Amphocin has been associated with the following:

- Shock
- Chills
- Fever
- Headache
- Changes in heartbeat
- Fast Breathing
- Fainting
- Blurred vision
- Nausea
- Vomiting
- Loss of appetite
- Pale skin
- Flushing
- Tiredness
- Diarrhea
- Stomach cramping

- ☠ Loss of appetite
- ☠ Heartburn
- ☠ Abnormal weight loss
- ☠ Muscle or joint pain
- ☠ Ringing in ears
- ☠ Hearing loss
- ☠ Pain, burning, numbness, or tingling in hands or feet
- ☠ Itching
- ☠ Hives
- ☠ Difficulty breathing or swallowing
- ☠ Wheezing
- ☠ Confusion
- ☠ Loss of consciousness or responsiveness
- ☠ Seizures
- ☠ Decreased urination
- ☠ Unusual bleeding or bruising
- ☠ Black or tarry stools
- ☠ Red blood in stools
- ☠ Bloody vomit
- ☠ Yellowing of eyes or skin
- ☠ Flu like symptoms
- ☠ Sore throat
- ☠ Cough
- ☠ High blood pressure
- ☠ Racing heart
- ☠ Abnormal liver function
- ☠ Cardiovascular changes
- ☠ Hemorrhage
- ☠ Confusion
- ☠ Dizziness
- ☠ Insomnia
- ☠ Tremor

- ☠ Thinking abnormality
- ☠ Anemia
- ☠ Edema
- ☠ Diarrhea
- ☠ Jaundice
- ☠ Coagulation disorder
- ☠ Asthma
- ☠ Rash
- ☠ Eye hemorrhage
- ☠ Blood in the urine (hematuria)

Tell your doctor and pharmacist what prescription and nonprescription medications, vitamins, nutritional supplements, and herbal products you are taking or plan to take.

Be sure to mention any of the following: aminoglycoside antibiotics such as amikacin (Amikin), gentamicin (Garamycin), kanamycin (Kantrex), neomycin (Nes-RX, Neo-Fradin), paramomycin (Humatin), streptomycin, and tobramycin (Tobi, Nebcin); certain antifungals such as clotrimazole, fluconazole, itraconazole (Sporanox), ketoconazole, and miconazole; corticotrophin (ACTH, H.P., Acthar Gel); cyclosporine (Neoral, Sandimmune); digoxin (Digitek, Lanoxicaps, Lanoxin); flucytosine (Ancobon); medications for the treatment of cancer, such as nitrogen

mustard; oral steroids such as dexamethasone (Decadron, Dexone), methylprednisolone (Medrol), and prednisone (Deltasone); and pentamidine (NebuPent, Pentam 300).

Tell your doctor if you are receiving transfusions or having radiation treatments. Also tell your doctor if you have or have ever had diabetes, or heart or kidney disease.

Tell your doctor if you are pregnant, or plan to become pregnant. If you become pregnant while taking Amphocin, call your doctor. Do not breastfeed if you are taking Amphocin.

If you are having surgery, including dental surgery, tell the doctor or dentist that you are taking Amphocin.

AMPHOTERICIN B

Amphotericin B can have serious side effects and should only be used for treatment of patients with progressive and potentially life-threatening fungal infections. It should not be used to treat noninvasive forms of fungal disease such as oral thrush, vaginal yeast infections, and esophageal yeast infections.

Amphotericin B is a generic drug sold under the brand names Amphocin and Fungizone.

Use of Amphotericin B has been associated with the following:

- Shock
- Chills
- Fever
- Headache
- Changes in heartbeat
- Fast Breathing
- Fainting
- Blurred vision
- Nausea
- Vomiting
- Loss of appetite
- Pale skin
- Flushing
- Tiredness

- ☠ Diarrhea
- ☠ Stomach cramping
- ☠ Loss of appetite
- ☠ Heartburn
- ☠ Abnormal weight loss
- ☠ Muscle or joint pain
- ☠ Ringing in ears
- ☠ Hearing loss
- ☠ Pain, burning, numbness, or tingling in hands or feet
- ☠ Itching
- ☠ Hives
- ☠ Difficulty breathing or swallowing
- ☠ Wheezing
- ☠ Confusion
- ☠ Loss of consciousness or responsiveness
- ☠ Seizures
- ☠ Decreased urination
- ☠ Unusual bleeding or bruising
- ☠ Black or tarry stools
- ☠ Red blood in stools
- ☠ Bloody vomit
- ☠ Yellowing of eyes or skin
- ☠ Flu like symptoms
- ☠ Sore throat
- ☠ Cough
- ☠ High blood pressure
- ☠ Racing heart
- ☠ Abnormal liver function
- ☠ Cardiovascular changes
- ☠ Hemorrhage
- ☠ Confusion
- ☠ Dizziness

- ☠ Insomnia
- ☠ Tremor
- ☠ Thinking abnormality
- ☠ Anemia
- ☠ Edema
- ☠ Diarrhea
- ☠ Jaundice
- ☠ Coagulation disorder
- ☠ Asthma
- ☠ Rash
- ☠ Eye hemorrhage
- ☠ Blood in the urine (hematuria)

Tell your doctor and pharmacist what prescription and nonprescription medications, vitamins, nutritional supplements, and herbal products you are taking or plan to take.

Be sure to mention any of the following: aminoglycoside antibiotics such as amikacin (Amikin), gentamicin (Garamycin), kanamycin (Kantrex), neomycin (Nes-RX, Neo-Fradin), paramomycin (Humatin), streptomycin, and tobramycin (Tobi, Nebcin); certain antifungals such as clotrimazole, fluconazole, itraconazole (Sporanox), ketoconazole, and miconazole; corticotrophin (ACTH, H.P., Acthar Gel); cyclosporine (Neoral, Sandimmune); digoxin (Digitek, Lanoxicaps, Lanoxin); flucytosine (Ancobon); medications for the treatment of cancer, such as nitrogen

mustard; oral steroids such as dexamethasone (Decadron, Dexone), methylprednisolone (Medrol), and prednisone (Deltasone); and pentamidine (NebuPent, Pentam 300).

Tell your doctor if you are receiving transfusions or having radiation treatments. Also tell your doctor if you have or have ever had diabetes, or heart or kidney disease.

Tell your doctor if you are pregnant, or plan to become pregnant. If you become pregnant while taking Amphotericin B, call your doctor. Do not breastfeed if you are taking Amphotericin B.

If you are having surgery, including dental surgery, tell the doctor or dentist that you are taking Amphotericin B.

Butoconazole

Butoconazole is used to treat yeast infections of the vagina. Butoconazole comes as a cream to insert into the vagina. It is usually used daily at bedtime for either 1 or 6 days.

Butoconazole is a generic drug sold under the brand names Femstat and Gynazole.

Butoconazole may cause the following side effects:

- Burning in vagina or urinary opening
- Irritation in vagina or urinary opening
- Pain in vagina or urinary opening
- Lower abdominal cramps
- Stomach pain
- Fever
- Chills
- Flu-like symptoms
- Foul-smelling discharge
- Rash
- Itching
- Swelling
- Severe Dizziness
- Trouble breathing

Butoconazole is for external use only. Do not let cream get into your eyes or mouth, and do not swallow it.

You should not use Butoconazole if you have a fever, abdominal pain, foul-smelling vaginal discharge, diabetes, HIV, or AIDS.

This medication may be harmful to an unborn baby. Tell your doctor if you are pregnant or plan to become pregnant during treatment.

Butoconazole contains mineral oil, which can weaken the latex rubber that condoms and diaphragms are made of. If you use either of these forms of birth control, they may not be as effective during your treatment with Butoconazole. Use another form of birth control while you are using Butoconazole and for at least 3 full days after your treatment has ended.

It is not known whether Butoconazole passes into breast milk or if it could harm a nursing baby. Do not use this medication without telling your doctor if you are breast-feeding a baby.

Avoid wearing tight-fitting, synthetic clothing such as nylon underwear or panty hose that does not allow air circulation. Wear loose-fitting clothing made of cotton and other natural fibers until your infection is healed.

Avoid using other vaginal creams or douches at the same time as Butoconazole vaginal unless your doctor approves.

Clotrimazole

Clotrimazole is prescribed to treat yeast infections of the vagina, mouth, and skin such as athlete's foot, jock itch, and body ringworm. It can also be used to prevent oral thrush in certain patients.

Clotrimazole is a generic drug sold under the brand names Lotrisone, Mycelex, Lotrimin, and Fem-Care.

Clotrimazole may cause the following side effects:

- Itching
- Burning
- Irritation
- Redness
- Swelling
- Stomach pain
- Fever
- Foul-smelling discharge if using the vaginal product
- Upset stomach or vomiting with the lozenges (troches)
- Extreme hair growth
- Skin thinning
- Skin discoloration
- Severe dizziness
- Trouble breathing

- ☠ Acne
- ☠ Stretch marks
- ☠ Hair bumps (folliculitis)
- ☠ Vision problems
- ☠ Persistent headache
- ☠ Increased thirst/urination
- ☠ Unusual weakness
- ☠ Sudden weight loss

Before using this medication, tell your doctor or pharmacist if you are allergic to clotrimazole or betamethasone; or to other azole antifungals (e.g., ketoconazole) or corticosteroids (e.g., triamcinolone); or if you have any other allergies.

Before using this medication, tell your doctor or pharmacist your medical history, especially of: immune system problems, poor blood circulation.

It is possible this medication will be absorbed into your bloodstream. This may have undesirable effects that may require additional corticosteroid treatment. Children and those using this drug for an extended time over most of the skin may be at higher risk, especially if they also have serious medical problems such as severe infections, injuries, or surgeries. This precaution applies for up to 1 year after stopping use of this drug.

Consult your doctor or pharmacist for more details, and tell them that you use (or have used) this medication.

Caution is advised when using this drug in the elderly because they may be more sensitive to the effects of the drug, especially thinning skin.

Caution is advised when using this drug in children because they may be more sensitive to the effects of too much steroid hormone. Though it is unlikely to occur with corticosteroids applied to the skin, this medication may affect growth in children if used for long periods. Monitor your child's height and rate of growth from time to time.

During pregnancy, this medication should be used only when clearly needed. Discuss the risks and benefits with your doctor.

It is not known whether this drug passes into breast milk when applied to the skin. Similar medications pass into breast milk when taken by mouth. Consult your doctor before breast-feeding.

Diflucan

Diflucan is used to treat fungal infections, including yeast infections of the vagina, mouth, throat, esophagus (tube leading from the mouth to the stomach), abdomen (area between the chest and waist), lungs, blood, and other organs. Diflucan is also used to treat meningitis (infection of the membranes covering the brain and spine) caused by fungus. Diflucan is also used to prevent yeast infections in patients who are likely to become infected because they are being treated with chemotherapy or radiation therapy before a bone marrow transplant (replacement of unhealthy spongy tissue inside the bones with healthy tissue). Diflucan is in a class of antifungals called triazoles. It works by slowing the growth of fungi that cause infection.

Diflucan is a brand name of the drug Fluconazole.

Use of Diflucan has been associated with liver (hepatic) injury, including death, in patients with serious underlying medical conditions.

Cases of severe reaction leading to skin loss (exfoliative disorder) have been recorded.

Approximately 26% of patients experience some adverse side effects from Diflucan including:

- Headache
- Dizziness
- Diarrhea
- Stomach pain
- Heartburn
- Change in ability to taste food
- Mistaking one taste for another
- Upset stomach
- Extreme tiredness
- Unusual bruising or bleeding
- Lack of energy
- Loss of appetite
- Pain in the upper right part of the stomach
- Yellowing of the skin or eyes
- Flu-like symptoms
- Dark urine
- Pale stools
- Seizures
- Rash
- Hives
- Itching
- Swelling of the face, throat, tongue, lips, eyes, hands, feet, ankles, or lower legs
- Difficulty breathing

- ☠ Difficulty swallowing
- ☠ Indigestion
- ☠ Nausea

Diflucan therapy has been associated with QT interval prolongation, which may lead to serious cardiac arrhythmias. Thus it is used with caution in patients with risk factors for prolonged QT interval such as electrolyte imbalance or use of other drugs which may prolong the QT interval (particularly cisapride).

High concentrations of Diflucan have been detected in human breast milk from patients receiving Diflucan therapy; it should not be used by breastfeeding mothers.

Tell your doctor and pharmacist if you are allergic to Diflucan, other antifungal medications such as itraconazole (Sporanox), ketoconazole (Nizoral), or voriconazole (Vfend) or any other, medications.

Do not take cisapride (Propulsid) while taking Diflucan.

Tell your doctor and pharmacist what prescription and nonprescription medications, vitamins, nutritional supplements, and herbal products you are taking, especially the following:

- Amiodarone (Cordarone)
- Anticoagulants (blood thinners) such as warfarin (Coumadin)
- Astemizole (Hismanal)
- Benzodiazepines such as midazolam (Versed)
- Cyclosporine (Neoral, Sandimmune)
- Disopyramide (Norpace)
- Diuretics (water pills) such as hydrochlorothiazide (HydroDIURIL, Microzide)
- Dofetilide (Tikosyn)
- Erythromycin (E.E.S, E-Mycin, Erythrocin)
- Isoniazid (INH, Nydrazid)
- Moxifloxacin (Avelox)
- Oral contraceptives (birth control pills)
- Oral medicine for diabetes such as glipizide (Glucotrol), glyburide (Diabeta, Micronase, Glycron, others), and tolbutamide (Orinase)
- Phenytoin (Dilantin)
- Pimozide (Orap)
- Procainamide (Procanbid, Pronestyl)
- Quinidine (Quinidex)
- Rifabutin (Mycobutin)
- Rifampin (Rifadin, Rimactane)

- Sotalolol (Betapace)
- Sparfloxacin (Zagam)
- Tacrolimus (Prograf)
- Terfenadine (Seldane)
- Theophylline (TheoDur)
- Thioridazine (Mellaril)
- Valproic acid (Depakene, Depakote)
- Zidovudine (Retrovir)

Tell your doctor if you drink or have ever drunk large amounts of alcohol and if you have or have ever had cancer; acquired immunodeficiency syndrome (AIDS); an irregular heartbeat; or heart, kidney or liver disease.

Tell your doctor if you are pregnant, plan to become pregnant, or are breast-feeding. If you become pregnant while taking Diflucan, call your doctor.

Symptoms of overdose may include:

- ☠ Hallucinations (seeing things or hearing voices that do not exist)
- ☠ Extreme fear that others are trying to harm you

Fem-Care

Fem-Care is prescribed to treat yeast infections of the vagina, mouth, and skin such as athlete's foot, jock itch, and body ringworm. It can also be used to prevent oral thrush in certain patients.

Fem-Care is a brand name for the drug Clotrimazole.

Fem-Care may cause the following side effects:

- Itching
- Burning
- Irritation
- Redness
- Swelling
- Stomach pain
- Fever
- Foul-smelling discharge if using the vaginal product
- Upset stomach or vomiting with the lozenges (troches)
- Extreme hair growth
- Skin thinning
- Skin discoloration
- Severe dizziness
- Trouble breathing
- Acne

- ☠ Stretch marks
- ☠ Hair bumps (folliculitis)
- ☠ Vision problems
- ☠ Persistent headache
- ☠ Increased thirst/urination
- ☠ Unusual weakness
- ☠ Sudden weight loss

Before using this medication, tell your doctor or pharmacist if you are allergic to clotrimazole or betamethasone; or to other azole antifungals (e.g., ketoconazole) or corticosteroids (e.g., triamcinolone); or if you have any other allergies.

Before using this medication, tell your doctor or pharmacist your medical history, especially of: immune system problems, poor blood circulation.

It is possible this medication will be absorbed into your bloodstream. This may have undesirable effects that may require additional corticosteroid treatment. Children and those using this drug for an extended time over most of the skin may be at higher risk, especially if they also have serious medical problems such as severe infections, injuries, or surgeries. This precaution applies for up to 1 year after stopping use of this drug.

Consult your doctor or pharmacist for more details, and tell them that you use (or have used) this medication.

Caution is advised when using this drug in the elderly because they may be more sensitive to the effects of the drug, especially thinning skin.

Caution is advised when using this drug in children because they may be more sensitive to the effects of too much steroid hormone. Though it is unlikely to occur with corticosteroids applied to the skin, this medication may affect growth in children if used for long periods. Monitor your child's height and rate of growth from time to time.

During pregnancy, this medication should be used only when clearly needed. Discuss the risks and benefits with your doctor.

It is not known whether this drug passes into breast milk when applied to the skin. Similar medications pass into breast milk when taken by mouth. Consult your doctor before breast-feeding.

Femizol

Femizol, an antifungal agent, is used for skin infections such as athlete's foot and jock itch and for vaginal yeast infections.

Femizol is a brand name for the generic drug Miconazole.

Femizol vaginal cream and suppositories are for use only in the vagina. These products are not to be taken by mouth. The vaginal suppositories are inserted, one per dose, in an applicator. Alternatively, the tube containing the vaginal cream is screwed onto the end of a special applicator tube, and the tube is then squeezed to fill the applicator. The patient then lies on her back with bent knees, inserts the applicator containing either the suppository or cream so that the tip of the applicator is high in the vagina, and then pushes the plunger in to deposit the suppository or cream into the vagina. The applicator should be washed with warm soap and water after each use.

Femizol usually is used once daily at bedtime. The 200 mg suppositories (Monistat 3) are inserted once nightly for 3 nights. The 100 mg suppositories

(Monistat-7) and intravaginal cream are inserted once nightly for 7 nights. The 1200 mg formulation (Monistat 1) is applied once for one night.

For fungal skin infections, the topical cream is applied as a thin layer to cover the affected skin and surrounding area, usually twice daily. The hands should be washed before and after application.

Femizol may cause the following side effects:

- Rash
- Burning at the site of application
- Itching
- Irritation of the skin or vagina
- Stomach pain
- Fever
- Foul-smelling vaginal discharge
- Diarrhea
- Vomiting
- Loss of appetite
- Hives
- Chills

There is very limited information on the use of Femizol during pregnancy. The physician must weigh the potential benefits against possible but unknown risks to the fetus.

It is not known if Femizol is secreted in breast milk in amounts that can affect the infant.

Tell your doctor about all the medicines you use (both prescription and nonprescription). Inform your doctor if you are taking:

- Anticoagulants (such as warfarin)
- Diabetes drugs
- Isoniazid
- Rifampin
- Rifabutin
- Phenytoin
- Cisapride

Femstat

Femstat is used to treat yeast infections of the vagina. Femstat comes as a cream to insert into the vagina. It is usually used daily at bedtime for either 1 or 6 days.

Femstat is a generic drug sold under the brand names Femstat and Gynazole.

Femstat may cause the following side effects:

- Burning in vagina or urinary opening
- Irritation in vagina or urinary opening
- Pain in vagina or urinary opening
- Lower abdominal cramps
- Stomach pain
- Fever
- Chills
- Flu-like symptoms
- Foul-smelling discharge
- Rash
- Itching
- Swelling
- Severe Dizziness
- Trouble breathing

Femstat is for external use only. Do not let cream get into your eyes or mouth, and do not swallow it.

You should not use Femstat vaginal if you have a fever, abdominal pain, foul-smelling vaginal discharge, diabetes, HIV, or AIDS.

This medication may be harmful to an unborn baby. Tell your doctor if you are pregnant or plan to become pregnant during treatment.

Femstat contains mineral oil, which can weaken the latex rubber that condoms and diaphragms are made of. If you use either of these forms of birth control, they may not be as effective during your treatment with Femstat. Use another form of birth control while you are using Femstat and for at least 3 full days after your treatment has ended.

It is not known whether Femstat passes into breast milk or if it could harm a nursing baby. Do not use this medication without telling your doctor if you are breast-feeding a baby.

Avoid wearing tight-fitting, synthetic clothing such as nylon underwear or panty hose that does not allow air circulation. Wear loose-fitting clothing made of cotton and other natural fibers until your infection is healed.

Avoid using other vaginal creams or douches at the same time as Femstat vaginal unless your doctor approves.

FLUCONAZOLE

Fluconazole is used to treat fungal infections, including yeast infections of the vagina, mouth, throat, esophagus (tube leading from the mouth to the stomach), abdomen (area between the chest and waist), lungs, blood, and other organs. Fluconazole is also used to treat meningitis (infection of the membranes covering the brain and spine) caused by fungus. Fluconazole is also used to prevent yeast infections in patients who are likely to become infected because they are being treated with chemotherapy or radiation therapy before a bone marrow transplant (replacement of unhealthy spongy tissue inside the bones with healthy tissue). Fluconazole is in a class of antifungals called triazoles. It works by slowing the growth of fungi that cause infection.

Fluconazole is a generic drug sold under the brand names Diflucan and Trican.

Use of Fluconazole has been associated with liver (hepatic) injury, including death, in patients with serious underlying medical conditions.

Cases of severe reaction leading to skin loss (exfoliative disorder) have been recorded.

Approximately 26% of patients experience some adverse side effects from Fluconazole including:

- Headache
- Dizziness
- Diarrhea
- Stomach pain
- Heartburn
- Change in ability to taste food
- Mistaking one taste for another
- Upset stomach
- Extreme tiredness
- Unusual bruising or bleeding
- Lack of energy
- Loss of appetite
- Pain in the upper right part of the stomach
- Yellowing of the skin or eyes
- Flu-like symptoms
- Dark urine
- Pale stools
- Seizures
- Rash
- Hives
- Itching
- Swelling of the face, throat, tongue, lips, eyes, hands, feet, ankles, or lower legs
- Difficulty breathing

- ☠ Difficulty swallowing
- ☠ Indigestion
- ☠ Nausea

Fluconazole therapy has been associated with QT interval prolongation, which may lead to serious cardiac arrhythmias. Thus it is used with caution in patients with risk factors for prolonged QT interval such as electrolyte imbalance or use of other drugs which may prolong the QT interval (particularly cisapride).

High concentrations of fluconazole have been detected in human breast milk from patients receiving fluconazole therapy; it should not be used by breastfeeding mothers.

Tell your doctor and pharmacist if you are allergic to fluconazole, other antifungal medications such as itraconazole (Sporanox), ketoconazole (Nizoral), or voriconazole (Vfend) or any other, medications.

Do not take cisapride (Propulsid) while taking fluconazole.

Tell your doctor and pharmacist what prescription and nonprescription medications, vitamins, nutritional supplements, and herbal products you are taking, especially the following:

- Amiodarone (Cordarone)

- Anticoagulants (blood thinners) such as warfarin (Coumadin)
- Astemizole (Hismanal)
- Benzodiazepines such as midazolam (Versed)
- Cyclosporine (Neoral, Sandimmune)
- Disopyramide (Norpace)
- Diuretics (water pills) such as hydrochlorothiazide (HydroDIURIL, Microzide)
- Dofetilide (Tikosyn)
- Erythromycin (E.E.S, E-Mycin, Erythrocin)
- Isoniazid (INH, Nydrazid)
- Moxifloxacin (Avelox)
- Oral contraceptives (birth control pills)
- Oral medicine for diabetes such as glipizide (Glucotrol), glyburide (Diabeta, Micronase, Glycron, others), and tolbutamide (Orinase)
- Phenytoin (Dilantin)
- Pimozide (Orap)
- Procainamide (Procanbid, Pronestyl)
- Quinidine (Quinidex)
- Rifabutin (Mycobutin)
- Rifampin (Rifadin, Rimactane)
- Sotalolol (Betapace)
- Sparfloxacin (Zagam)

- Tacrolimus (Prograf)
- Terfenadine (Seldane)
- Theophylline (TheoDur)
- Thioridazine (Mellaril)
- Valproic acid (Depakene, Depakote)
- Zidovudine (Retrovir)

Tell your doctor if you drink or have ever drunk large amounts of alcohol and if you have or have ever had cancer; acquired immunodeficiency syndrome (AIDS); an irregular heartbeat; or heart, kidney or liver disease.

Tell your doctor if you are pregnant, plan to become pregnant, or are breast-feeding. If you become pregnant while taking fluconazole, call your doctor.

Symptoms of overdose may include:

- ☠ Hallucinations (seeing things or hearing voices that do not exist)
- ☠ Extreme fear that others are trying to harm you

Fulvicin

Fulvicin is prescribed to treat skin infections such as jock itch, athlete's foot, and ringworm; and fungal infections of the scalp, fingernails, and toenails.

Fulvicin comes as a tablet, capsule, and liquid to take by mouth. It is usually taken once a day or can be taken two to four times a day. Although your symptoms may get better in a few days, you will have to take Fulvicin for a long time before the infection is completely gone. It is usually taken for 2 to 4 weeks for skin infections, 4 to 6 weeks for hair and scalp infections, 4 to 8 weeks for foot infections, 3 to 4 months for fingernail infections, and at least 6 months for toenail infections.

Fulvicin is a brand name for the drug Griseofulvin.

Use of Fulvicin has been associated with:

- Nausea
- Gastric distress
- Abdominal cramps
- Vomiting
- Diarrhea
- Allergic reactions

- ☠ Chest pain
- ☠ Dryness of the mouth
- ☠ Muscle and joint aches and pains
- ☠ Fever
- ☠ Changes in blood coagulation
- ☠ Decrease in the production of blood cells
- ☠ Thirst
- ☠ Fatigue
- ☠ Dizziness
- ☠ Faintness
- ☠ Sore throat
- ☠ Skin rash
- ☠ Mouth sores

Tell your doctor and pharmacist what prescription and nonprescription medications you are taking, especially anticoagulants ('blood thinners') such as warfarin (Coumadin), oral contraceptives, cyclosporine (Neoral, Sandimmune), Phenobarbital (Luminal), and vitamins.

Tell your doctor if you have or have ever had liver disease, porphyria, lupus, or a history of alcohol abuse.

Tell your doctor if you are pregnant, plan to become pregnant, or are breast-feeding. If you become pregnant while taking Fulvicin, call your doctor.

Tell your doctor if you drink alcohol.

Fulvicin may make your skin sensitive to sunlight. You should avoid unnecessary or prolonged exposure to sunlight and wear protective clothing, sunglasses, and sunscreen.

Fungizone

Fungizone can have serious side effects and should only be used for treatment of patients with progressive and potentially life-threatening fungal infections. It should not be used to treat noninvasive forms of fungal disease such as oral thrush, vaginal yeast infections, and esophageal yeast infections.

Fungizone is a brand name for the drug Amphotericin B.

Use of Amphotericin has been associated with the following:

- Shock
- Chills
- Fever
- Headache
- Changes in heartbeat
- Fast Breathing
- Fainting
- Blurred vision
- Nausea
- Vomiting
- Loss of appetite
- Pale skin
- Flushing
- Tiredness
- Diarrhea

- ☠ Stomach cramping
- ☠ Loss of appetite
- ☠ Heartburn
- ☠ Abnormal weight loss
- ☠ Muscle or joint pain
- ☠ Ringing in ears
- ☠ Hearing loss
- ☠ Pain, burning, numbness, or tingling in hands or feet
- ☠ Itching
- ☠ Hives
- ☠ Difficulty breathing or swallowing
- ☠ Wheezing
- ☠ Confusion
- ☠ Loss of consciousness or responsiveness
- ☠ Seizures
- ☠ Decreased urination
- ☠ Unusual bleeding or bruising
- ☠ Black or tarry stools
- ☠ Red blood in stools
- ☠ Bloody vomit
- ☠ Yellowing of eyes or skin
- ☠ Flu like symptoms
- ☠ Sore throat
- ☠ Cough
- ☠ High blood pressure
- ☠ Racing heart
- ☠ Abnormal liver function
- ☠ Cardiovascular changes
- ☠ Hemorrhage
- ☠ Confusion
- ☠ Dizziness
- ☠ Insomnia

- ☠ Tremor
- ☠ Thinking abnormality
- ☠ Anemia
- ☠ Edema
- ☠ Diarrhea
- ☠ Jaundice
- ☠ Coagulation disorder
- ☠ Asthma
- ☠ Rash
- ☠ Eye hemorrhage
- ☠ Blood in the urine (hematuria)

Tell your doctor and pharmacist what prescription and nonprescription medications, vitamins, nutritional supplements, and herbal products you are taking or plan to take.

Be sure to mention any of the following: aminoglycoside antibiotics such as amikacin (Amikin), gentamicin (Garamycin), kanamycin (Kantrex), neomycin (Nes-RX, Neo-Fradin), paramomycin (Humatin), streptomycin, and tobramycin (Tobi, Nebcin); certain antifungals such as clotrimazole, fluconazole, itraconazole (Sporanox), ketoconazole, and miconazole; corticotrophin (ACTH, H.P., Acthar Gel); cyclosporine (Neoral, Sandimmune); digoxin (Digitek, Lanoxicaps, Lanoxin); flucytosine (Ancobon); medications for the treatment of cancer, such as nitrogen

mustard; oral steroids such as dexamethasone (Decadron, Dexone), methylprednisolone (Medrol), and prednisone (Deltasone); and pentamidine (NebuPent, Pentam 300).

Tell your doctor if you are receiving transfusions or having radiation treatments. Also tell your doctor if you have or have ever had diabetes, or heart or kidney disease.

Tell your doctor if you are pregnant, or plan to become pregnant. If you become pregnant while taking Fungizone, call your doctor. Do not breastfeed if you are taking Fungizone.

If you are having surgery, including dental surgery, tell the doctor or dentist that you are taking Fungizone.

Fungoid

Fungoid, an antifungal agent, is used for skin infections such as athlete's foot and jock itch and for vaginal yeast infections.

Fungoid is a brand name for the generic drug Miconazole.

Fungoid vaginal cream and suppositories are for use only in the vagina. These products are not to be taken by mouth. The vaginal suppositories are inserted, one per dose, in an applicator. Alternatively, the tube containing the vaginal cream is screwed onto the end of a special applicator tube, and the tube is then squeezed to fill the applicator. The patient then lies on her back with bent knees, inserts the applicator containing either the suppository or cream so that the tip of the applicator is high in the vagina, and then pushes the plunger in to deposit the suppository or cream into the vagina. The applicator should be washed with warm soap and water after each use.

Fungoid usually is used once daily at bedtime. The 200 mg suppositories (Monistat 3) are inserted once nightly for 3 nights. The100 mg suppositories

(Monistat-7) and intravaginal cream are inserted once nightly for 7 nights. The 1200 mg formulation (Monistat 1) is applied once for one night.

For fungal skin infections, the topical cream is applied as a thin layer to cover the affected skin and surrounding area, usually twice daily. The hands should be washed before and after application.

Fungoid may cause the following side effects:

- Rash
- Burning at the site of application
- Itching
- Irritation of the skin or vagina
- Stomach pain
- Fever
- Foul-smelling vaginal discharge
- Diarrhea
- Vomiting
- Loss of appetite
- Hives
- Chills

There is very limited information on the use of Fungoid during pregnancy. The physician must weigh the potential benefits against possible but unknown risks to the fetus.

It is not known if Fungoid is secreted in breast milk in amounts that can affect the infant.

Tell your doctor about all the medicines you use (both prescription and nonprescription). Inform your doctor if you are taking:

- Anticoagulants (such as warfarin)
- Diabetes drugs
- Isoniazid
- Rifampin
- Rifabutin
- Phenytoin
- Cisapride

Grifulvin

Grifulvin is prescribed to treat skin infections such as jock itch, athlete's foot, and ringworm; and fungal infections of the scalp, fingernails, and toenails.

Grifulvin comes as a tablet, capsule, and liquid to take by mouth. It is usually taken once a day or can be taken two to four times a day. Although your symptoms may get better in a few days, you will have to take Grifulvin for a long time before the infection is completely gone. It is usually taken for 2 to 4 weeks for skin infections, 4 to 6 weeks for hair and scalp infections, 4 to 8 weeks for foot infections, 3 to 4 months for fingernail infections, and at least 6 months for toenail infections.

Grifulvin is a brand name for the drug Griseofulvin.

Use of Grifulvin has been associated with:

- Nausea
- Gastric distress
- Abdominal cramps
- Vomiting

- ☠ Diarrhea
- ☠ Allergic reactions
- ☠ Chest pain
- ☠ Dryness of the mouth
- ☠ Muscle and joint aches and pains
- ☠ Fever
- ☠ Changes in blood coagulation
- ☠ Decrease in the production of blood cells
- ☠ Thirst
- ☠ Fatigue
- ☠ Dizziness
- ☠ Faintness
- ☠ Sore throat
- ☠ Skin rash
- ☠ Mouth sores

Tell your doctor and pharmacist what prescription and nonprescription medications you are taking, especially anticoagulants ('blood thinners') such as warfarin (Coumadin), oral contraceptives, cyclosporine (Neoral, Sandimmune), Phenobarbital (Luminal), and vitamins.

Tell your doctor if you have or have ever had liver disease, porphyria, lupus, or a history of alcohol abuse.

Tell your doctor if you are pregnant, plan to become pregnant, or are breast-feeding. If you become pregnant while taking Grifulvin, call your doctor.

Tell your doctor if you drink alcohol.

Grifulvin may make your skin sensitive to sunlight. You should avoid unnecessary or prolonged exposure to sunlight and wear protective clothing, sunglasses, and sunscreen.

GRISEOFULVIN

Griseofulvin is prescribed to treat skin infections such as jock itch, athlete's foot, and ringworm; and fungal infections of the scalp, fingernails, and toenails.

Griseofulvin comes as a tablet, capsule, and liquid to take by mouth. It is usually taken once a day or can be taken two to four times a day. Although your symptoms may get better in a few days, you will have to take Griseofulvin for a long time before the infection is completely gone. It is usually taken for 2 to 4 weeks for skin infections, 4 to 6 weeks for hair and scalp infections, 4 to 8 weeks for foot infections, 3 to 4 months for fingernail infections, and at least 6 months for toenail infections.

Griseofulvin is a generic drug sold under the brand names Fulvicin, Grifulvin, and Gris-PEG.

Use of Griseofulvin has been associated with:

- Nausea
- Gastric distress
- Abdominal cramps
- Vomiting

- ☠ Diarrhea
- ☠ Allergic reactions
- ☠ Chest pain
- ☠ Dryness of the mouth
- ☠ Muscle and joint aches and pains
- ☠ Fever
- ☠ Changes in blood coagulation
- ☠ Decrease in the production of blood cells
- ☠ Thirst
- ☠ Fatigue
- ☠ Dizziness
- ☠ Faintness
- ☠ Sore throat
- ☠ Skin rash
- ☠ Mouth sores

Tell your doctor and pharmacist what prescription and nonprescription medications you are taking, especially anticoagulants ('blood thinners') such as warfarin (Coumadin), oral contraceptives, cyclosporine (Neoral, Sandimmune), Phenobarbital (Luminal), and vitamins.

Tell your doctor if you have or have ever had liver disease, porphyria, lupus, or a history of alcohol abuse.

Tell your doctor if you are pregnant, plan to become pregnant, or are breast-feeding. If you become pregnant while taking Griseofulvin, call your doctor.

Tell your doctor if you drink alcohol.

Griseofulvin may make your skin sensitive to sunlight. You should avoid unnecessary or prolonged exposure to sunlight and wear protective clothing, sunglasses, and sunscreen.

Gris-PEG

Gris-PEG is prescribed to treat skin infections such as jock itch, athlete's foot, and ringworm; and fungal infections of the scalp, fingernails, and toenails.

Gris-PEG comes as a tablet, capsule, and liquid to take by mouth. It is usually taken once a day or can be taken two to four times a day. Although your symptoms may get better in a few days, you will have to take Gris-PEG for a long time before the infection is completely gone. It is usually taken for 2 to 4 weeks for skin infections, 4 to 6 weeks for hair and scalp infections, 4 to 8 weeks for foot infections, 3 to 4 months for fingernail infections, and at least 6 months for toenail infections.

Gris-PEG is a brand name for the drug Griseofulvin.

Use of Gris-PEG has been associated with:

- Nausea
- Gastric distress
- Abdominal cramps
- Vomiting
- Diarrhea

- ☠ Allergic reactions
- ☠ Chest pain
- ☠ Dryness of the mouth
- ☠ Muscle and joint aches and pains
- ☠ Fever
- ☠ Changes in blood coagulation
- ☠ Decrease in the production of blood cells
- ☠ Thirst
- ☠ Fatigue
- ☠ Dizziness
- ☠ Faintness
- ☠ Sore throat
- ☠ Skin rash
- ☠ Mouth sores

Tell your doctor and pharmacist what prescription and nonprescription medications you are taking, especially anticoagulants ('blood thinners') such as warfarin (Coumadin), oral contraceptives, cyclosporine (Neoral, Sandimmune), Phenobarbital (Luminal), and vitamins.

Tell your doctor if you have or have ever had liver disease, porphyria, lupus, or a history of alcohol abuse.

Tell your doctor if you are pregnant, plan to become pregnant, or are breast-feeding. If you become pregnant while taking Gris-PEG, call your doctor.

Tell your doctor if you drink alcohol.

Gris-PEG may make your skin sensitive to sunlight. You should avoid unnecessary or prolonged exposure to sunlight and wear protective clothing, sunglasses, and sunscreen.

Gynazole

Gynazole is used to treat yeast infections of the vagina. Gynazole comes as a cream to insert into the vagina. It is usually used daily at bedtime for either 1 or 6 days.

Gynazole is a generic drug sold under the brand names Femstat and Gynazole.

Gynazole may cause the following side effects:

- Burning in vagina or urinary opening
- Irritation in vagina or urinary opening
- Pain in vagina or urinary opening
- Lower abdominal cramps
- Stomach pain
- Fever
- Chills
- Flu-like symptoms
- Foul-smelling discharge
- Rash
- Itching
- Swelling
- Severe Dizziness
- Trouble breathing

Gynazole is for external use only. Do not let cream get into your eyes or mouth, and do not swallow it.

You should not use Gynazole vaginal if you have a fever, abdominal pain, foul-smelling vaginal discharge, diabetes, HIV, or AIDS.

This medication may be harmful to an unborn baby. Tell your doctor if you are pregnant or plan to become pregnant during treatment.

Gynazole contains mineral oil, which can weaken the latex rubber that condoms and diaphragms are made of. If you use either of these forms of birth control, they may not be as effective during your treatment with Gynazole. Use another form of birth control while you are using Gynazole and for at least 3 full days after your treatment has ended.

It is not known whether Gynazole passes into breast milk or if it could harm a nursing baby. Do not use this medication without telling your doctor if you are breast-feeding a baby.

Avoid wearing tight-fitting, synthetic clothing such as nylon underwear or panty hose that does not allow air circulation. Wear loose-fitting clothing made of cotton and other natural fibers until your infection is healed.

Avoid using other vaginal creams or douches at the same time as Gynazole vaginal unless your doctor approves.

ITRACONAZOLE

Itraconazole capsules are prescribed to treat fungal infections that begin in the lungs and can spread through the body. Itraconazole capsules are also used to treat fungal infections of the fingernails and/or toenails. Itraconazole oral solution is used to treat yeast infections of the mouth and throat and suspected fungal infections in patients with fever and certain other signs of infection. Itraconazole is in a class of antifungals called triazoles. It works by slowing the growth of fungi that cause infection.

Itraconazole is a generic drug sold under the brand name Sporanox.

Itraconazole can cause congestive heart failure (condition in which the heart cannot pump enough blood through the body).

Tell your doctor if you have or have ever had heart failure; a heart attack; an irregular heartbeat; any other type of heart disease; lung, liver, or kidney disease; or any other serious health problem.

If you experience any of the following symptoms, stop taking itraconazole and, call your doctor immediately:

- Shortness of breath
- Coughing up white or pink phlegm
- Weakness
- Excessive tiredness
- Fast heartbeat
- Swelling of the feet, ankles, or legs
- Sudden weight gain

People who take itraconazole may experience the following side effects:

- Diarrhea or loose stools
- Constipation
- Gas
- Stomach pain
- Heartburn
- Sore or bleeding gums
- Sores in or around the mouth
- Headache
- Dizziness
- Sweating
- Muscle pain
- Decreased sexual desire or ability
- Nervousness
- Depression
- Runny nose and other cold symptoms
- Unusual dreams
- Excessive tiredness
- Loss of appetite

- ☠ Upset stomach
- ☠ Vomiting
- ☠ Yellowing of the skin or eyes
- ☠ Dark urine
- ☠ Pale stools
- ☠ Tingling or numbness of the hands or feet
- ☠ Fever, chills, or other signs of infection
- ☠ Frequent or painful urination
- ☠ Shaking hands that you cannot control
- ☠ Rash
- ☠ Hives
- ☠ Itching
- ☠ Difficulty breathing or swallowing

Use of Itraconazole has been associated with serious hepatotoxicity, including liver failure and death. Some of these cases occurred within the first week of use.

Life-threatening irregularities in heart rhythms (cardiac dysrhythmias), and sudden death have occurred when patients were using medications in addition to Itraconazole, such as Quinidine. Cases of congestive heart failure and pulmonary edema have also been experienced.

Do not take the following medications while you are taking Itraconazole. If you do you may experience serious irregular heartbeats:

- Cisapride (Propulsid)
- Dofetilide (Tikosyn)
- Pimozide (Orap)
- Quinidine (Quinaglute, Quinidex, others)

Talk to your doctor about the risks of taking itraconazole.

Tell your doctor and pharmacist if you are allergic to Itraconazole; other antifungal medications such as fluconazole (Diflucan), ketoconazole (Nizoral), or voriconazole (Vfend); or any other medications.

If you are taking itraconazole oral solution, tell your doctor if you are allergic to saccharin or sulfa medications.

Do not take itraconazole if you are taking any of the following medications:

- Ergot-type medications such as dihydroergotamine (D.H.E. 45, Migranal)
- Ergoloid mesylates (Germinal, Hydergine)
- Ergonovine (Ergotrate)
- Ergotamine (Bellergal-S, Cafergot, Ergomar, Wigraine)

- Methylergonovine (Methergine)
- Methysergide (Sansert)
- Lovastatin (Mevacor)
- Simvastatin (Zocor)
- Triazolam (Halcion)

Tell your doctor and pharmacist what other prescription and nonprescription medications, vitamins, nutritional supplements and herbal products you are taking, especially:

- Alfentanil (Alfenta)
- Alprazolam (Xanax)
- Anticoagulants (blood thinners) such as warfarin (Coumadin)
- Atorvastatin (Lipitor)
- Buspirone (BuSpar)
- Busulfan (Myleran)
- Calcium channel blockers such as amlodipine (Norvasc), felodipine (Plendil), isradipine (Dynacirc), nifedipine (Adalat, Procardia) nicardipine (Cardene) nimodipine (Nimotop), nisoldipine (Sular), and verapamil (Calan, Covera, Isoptin, Verelan)
- Carbamazepine (Tegretol)

- Cerivastatin (Baycol) (not available in the United States)
- Cilostazol (Pletal)
- Clarithromycin (Biaxin)
- Cyclosporine (Neoral, Sandimmune)
- Diazepam (Valium)
- Digoxin (Lanoxin)
- Disopyramide (Norpace)
- Docetaxel (Taxotere)
- Eletriptan (Relpax)
- Erythromycin (E.E.S., Erythrocin, E-Mycin)
- Halofantrine (Halfan)
- HIV protease inhibitors such as indinavir (Crixivan), ritonavir (Norvir), and saquinavir (Fortovase, Invirase)
- Isoniazid (INH, Nydrazid)
- Medications for erectile dysfunction such as sildenafil (Viagra), tadalafil (Cialis), and vardenafil (Levitra)
- Midazolam (Versed)
- Nevirapine (Viramune)
- Oral contraceptives (birth control pills)
- Oral medicine for diabetes
- Phenobarbital (Luminal, Solfoton)
- Phenytoin (Dilantin)
- Rifabutin (Mycobutin)

- Rifampin (Rifadin, Rimactane)
- Sirolimus (Rapamune)
- Steroids such as dexamethasone (Decadron), budesonide (Entocort EC), and methylprednisolone (Medrol)
- Tacrolimus (Prograf)
- Trimetrexate (Neutrexin)
- Vinblastine (Velban)
- Vincristine (Oncovin)
- Vinorelbine (Navelbine)

Many other medications may also interact with Itraconazole, so be sure to tell your doctor about all the medications you are taking, even those that do not appear on this list.

You should know that Itraconazole may remain in your body for several months after you stop taking it. Tell your doctor that you have recently stopped taking Itraconazole before you start taking any other medications during the first few months after your treatment.

If you are taking an antacid, take it 1 hour before or 2 hours after you take Itraconazole.
Tell your doctor if you have or have ever had AIDS, cystic fibrosis (an inborn disease that causes problems with

breathing, digestion, and reproduction), or any condition that decreases the amount of acid in your stomach.

Tell your doctor if you are pregnant, plan to become pregnant, or are breast-feeding. You should not take Itraconazole to treat nail fungus if you are pregnant or could become pregnant. You may start to take Itraconazole to treat nail fungus only on the second or third day of your menstrual period when you are sure you are not pregnant. You must use effective birth control during your treatment and for 2 months afterward. If you become pregnant while taking Itraconazole to treat any condition, call your doctor immediately.

One of the ingredients in itraconazole oral solution caused cancer in some types of laboratory animals. It is not known whether people who take itraconazole solution have an increased risk of developing cancer. Talk to your doctor about the risks of taking itraconazole solution.

KETOCONAZOLE

Ketoconazole is prescribed to treat fungal infections. Ketoconazole is most often used to treat fungal infections that can spread to different parts of the body through the bloodstream such as yeast infections of the mouth, skin, urinary tract, and blood, and certain fungal infections that begin on the skin or in the lungs and can spread through the body. Ketoconazole is also used to treat fungal infections of the skin or nails that cannot be treated with other medications. Ketoconazole is in a class of antifungals called imidazoles. It works by slowing the growth of fungi that cause infection.

Ketoconazole is a generic drug sole under the brand name Nizoral.

Use of Ketoconazole has been associated with the following:

- ☠ Hepatotoxicity
- ☠ Headache
- ☠ Dizziness
- ☠ Tremors
- ☠ Nervousness
- ☠ Rash
- ☠ Swelling of the breasts
- ☠ Diarrhea

- ☠ Rectal bleeding
- ☠ Anemia
- ☠ Shock
- ☠ Cataract enlargement
- ☠ Shortness of breath
- ☠ Nausea
- ☠ Vomiting
- ☠ Abdominal pain
- ☠ Heartburn
- ☠ Extreme tiredness
- ☠ Loss of appetite
- ☠ Yellowing of skin or eyes
- ☠ Dark yellow urine
- ☠ Pale stools
- ☠ Pain in upper right part of stomach
- ☠ Flu-like symptoms

Ketoconazole may cause liver damage and should not be taken with:

- Acetaminophen (Tylenol, others)
- Cholesterol-lowering medications (statins) such as Atorvastatin (Lipitor), fluvastatin (Lescol), Lovastatin (Mevacor), pravastatin (Pravachol), or Simvastatin (Zocor)
- Isoniazid (INH, Nydrazid)
- Methotrexate (Rheumatrex)
- Niacin (nicotinic acid)
- Rifampin
- Astemizole (Hismanal)

- Cisapride (Propulsid)
- Terfenadine (Seldane)

Tell your doctor and pharmacist what other prescription and nonprescription medications, vitamins, nutritional supplements, and herbal products you are taking. Including any of the following:

- Alprazolam (Xanax)
- Anticoagulants ('blood thinners') such as warfarin (Coumadin)
- Buspirone (Buspar)
- Calcium channel blockers such as amlodipine (Norvasc), diltiazem (Cardizem, Dilacor, Tiazac), felodipine (Plendil), nifedipine (Adalat, Procardia), nisoldipine (Sular), and verapamil (Calan, Covera, Isoptin, Verelan)
- Clarithromycin (Biaxin)
- Cyclosporine (Neoral, Sandimmune)
- Diazepam (Valium)
- Digoxin (Lanoxin)
- Erythromycin (E.E.S., E-Mycin, Erythrocin)
- HIV protease inhibitors such as indinavir (Crixivan), ritonavir (Norvir), and

saquinavir (Invirase, Fortovase)
- Loratadine (Claritin)
- Medications for diabetes
- Medications for erectile dysfunction such as sildenafil (Viagra), tadalafil (Cialis) and vardenafil (Levitra)
- Methadone (Dolophine)
- Methylprednisolone (Medrol)
- Midazolam (Versed)
- Phenytoin (Dilantin)
- Pimozide (Orap)
- Quinidine (Quinidex, Quinaglute)
- Quinine
- Tacrolimus (Prograf)
- Tamoxifen (Nolvadex)
- Telithromycin (Ketek)
- Trazodone (Desyrel)
- Vincristine (Vincasar).

Your doctor may need to change the doses of your medications or monitor you carefully for side effects.

if you are taking antacids; antihistamines; medications for heartburn or ulcers such as cimetidine (Tagamet), famotidine (Pepcid), nizatadine (Axid), or ranitidine (Zantac); or medications for irritable bowel disease, motion sickness, Parkinson's disease, ulcers, or urinary problems, take them 2 hours after you take ketoconazole.

Tell your doctor if you are pregnant, plan to become pregnant, or are breast-feeding. If you become pregnant while taking ketoconazole, call your doctor. Do not breastfeed while you are taking ketoconazole.

Ask your doctor about the safe use of alcoholic beverages while you are taking ketoconazole. You may experience unpleasant symptoms such as flushing, rash, upset stomach, headache, and swelling of the hands, feet, ankles, or lower legs if you drink alcohol while you are taking ketoconazole.

Keep all appointments with your doctor and the laboratory. Your doctor will order certain tests to check your body's response to Ketoconazole.

LAMISIL

Lamisil is used to treat fungal infections of the toenail and fingernail. Lamisil is in a class of medications called antifungals. It works by stopping the growth of fungi. Lamisil comes as a tablet to take by mouth. It is usually taken once a day for 6 weeks for fingernail fungus and once a day for 12 weeks for toenail fungus. Follow the directions on your prescription label carefully, and ask your doctor or pharmacist to explain any part you do not understand. Take Lamisil exactly as directed. Do not take more or less of it or take it more often than prescribed by your doctor.

Lamisil is a brand name of the drug Terbinafine.

Use of Lamisil has been associated with the following:

- Liver failure, leading to liver transplant or death
- Serious skin reactions
- Serious blood disorders
- Rash
- Eczema
- Itch
- Diarrhea

- ☠ Abdominal pain
- ☠ Nausea
- ☠ Vomiting
- ☠ Headache
- ☠ Fatigue
- ☠ Muscle and joint pain
- ☠ Hypoglycemia
- ☠ Change in taste or loss of taste
- ☠ Hives
- ☠ Loss of appetite
- ☠ Vomiting
- ☠ Extreme tiredness
- ☠ Pain in the right upper part of stomach
- ☠ Dark urine
- ☠ Pale stools
- ☠ Fever
- ☠ Sore throat

Tell your doctor and pharmacist what prescription and nonprescription medications, vitamins, nutritional supplements, and herbal products you are taking.

Be sure to mention any of the following:

- Anticoagulants (blood thinners) such as warfarin (Coumadin)
- Antidepressants such as amitriptyline (Elavil), amoxapine (Asendin), clomipramine (Anafranil),

desipramine (Norpramin), doxepin (Adapin, Sinequan), imipramine (Tofranil), nortriptyline (Aventyl, Pamelor), protriptyline (Vivactil), and trimipramine (Surmontil)
- Beta-blockers such as atenolol (Tenormin), labetalol (Normodyne), metoprolol (Lopressor, Toprol XL), nadolol (Corgard), and propranolol (Inderal)
- Cimetidine (Tagamet)
- Medications that suppress the immune system such as azathioprine (Imuran), cyclosporine (Neoral, Sandimmune), methotrexate (Rheumatrex), sirolimus (Rapamune), and tacrolimus (Prograf)
- Rifampin (Rifadin, Rimactane); and selegiline (Eldepryl)

If you use any of the above drugs your doctor may need to change the doses of your medications or monitor you carefully for side effects.

Tell your doctor if you have or have ever had kidney or liver disease, human immunodeficiency virus (HIV), or acquired immunodeficiency syndrome (AIDS).

Tell your doctor if you are pregnant, plan to become pregnant, or are breast-feeding. If you become pregnant while taking Lamisil, call your doctor immediately. You should not take Lamisil while breast-feeding.

Terconazole

Terconazole is used to treat fungal and yeast infections of the vagina. Terconazole comes as a cream and suppository to insert into the vagina. It is usually used daily at bedtime for either 3 or 7 days. Always follow the directions on your prescription label carefully, and ask your doctor or pharmacist to explain any part you do not understand. Use terconazole exactly as directed. Do not use more or less of it or use it more often than prescribed by your doctor.

Terconazole is available under the brand name Terazol.

Terconazole may cause these side effects:

- Headache
- Missed menstrual periods
- Burning in vagina
- Irritation in vagina
- Stomach pain
- Fever
- Chills
- Flu-like symptoms
- Foul-smelling vaginal discharge

Terconazole is for external use only. Do not let cream get into your eyes or mouth, and do not swallow it.

Refrain from sexual intercourse. An ingredient in the cream may weaken certain latex products like condoms or diaphragms; do not use such products within 72 hours of using this medication. Wear clean cotton panties (or panties with cotton crotches), not panties made of nylon, rayon, or other synthetic fabrics.

It is not known whether this drug is excreted in human milk. Animal studies have shown that offspring exposed via mother's milk of showed decreased survival during the first few post-partum days. Because many drugs are excreted in human milk, and because of the potential for adverse reaction in nursing infants from Terconazole, a decision should be made whether to discontinue nursing or to discontinue the drug, taking into account the importance of the drug to the mother.

Lotrimin

Lotrimin, an antifungal agent, is used for skin infections such as athlete's foot and jock itch and for vaginal yeast infections.

Lotrimin is a brand name for the generic drug Miconazole.

Lotrimin vaginal cream and suppositories are for use only in the vagina. These products are not to be taken by mouth. The vaginal suppositories are inserted, one per dose, in an applicator. Alternatively, the tube containing the vaginal cream is screwed onto the end of a special applicator tube, and the tube is then squeezed to fill the applicator. The patient then lies on her back with bent knees, inserts the applicator containing either the suppository or cream so that the tip of the applicator is high in the vagina, and then pushes the plunger in to deposit the suppository or cream into the vagina. The applicator should be washed with warm soap and water after each use.

Lotrimin usually is used once daily at bedtime. The 200 mg suppositories (Monistat 3) are inserted once nightly for 3 nights. The 100 mg suppositories

(Monistat-7) and intravaginal cream are inserted once nightly for 7 nights. The 1200 mg formulation (Monistat 1) is applied once for one night.

For fungal skin infections, the topical cream is applied as a thin layer to cover the affected skin and surrounding area, usually twice daily. The hands should be washed before and after application.

Lotrimin may cause the following side effects:

- Rash
- Burning at the site of application
- Itching
- Irritation of the skin or vagina
- Stomach pain
- Fever
- Foul-smelling vaginal discharge
- Diarrhea
- Vomiting
- Loss of appetite
- Hives
- Chills

There is very limited information on the use of Lotrimin during pregnancy. The physician must weigh the potential benefits against possible but unknown risks to the fetus.

It is not known if Lotrimin is secreted in breast milk in amounts that can affect the infant.

Tell your doctor about all the medicines you use (both prescription and nonprescription). Inform your doctor if you are taking:

- Anticoagulants (such as warfarin)
- Diabetes drugs
- Isoniazid
- Rifampin
- Rifabutin
- Phenytoin
- Cisapride

Lotrisone

Lotrisone is prescribed to treat yeast infections of the vagina, mouth, and skin such as athlete's foot, jock itch, and body ringworm. It can also be used to prevent oral thrush in certain patients.

Lotrisone is a brand name for the drug Clotrimazole.

Lotrisone may cause the following side effects:

- Itching
- Burning
- Irritation
- Redness
- Swelling
- Stomach pain
- Fever
- Foul-smelling discharge if using the vaginal product
- Upset stomach or vomiting with the lozenges (troches)
- Extreme hair growth
- Skin thinning
- Skin discoloration
- Severe dizziness
- Trouble breathing
- Acne
- Stretch marks

- ☠ Hair bumps (folliculitis)
- ☠ Vision problems
- ☠ Persistent headache
- ☠ Increased thirst/urination
- ☠ Unusual weakness
- ☠ Sudden weight loss

Before using this medication, tell your doctor or pharmacist if you are allergic to clotrimazole or betamethasone; or to other azole antifungals (e.g., ketoconazole) or corticosteroids (e.g., triamcinolone); or if you have any other allergies.

Before using this medication, tell your doctor or pharmacist your medical history, especially of: immune system problems, poor blood circulation.

It is possible this medication will be absorbed into your bloodstream. This may have undesirable effects that may require additional corticosteroid treatment. Children and those using this drug for an extended time over most of the skin may be at higher risk, especially if they also have serious medical problems such as severe infections, injuries, or surgeries. This precaution applies for up to 1 year after stopping use of this drug.

Consult your doctor or pharmacist for more details, and tell them that you use (or have used) this medication.

Caution is advised when using this drug in the elderly because they may be more sensitive to the effects of the drug, especially thinning skin.

Caution is advised when using this drug in children because they may be more sensitive to the effects of too much steroid hormone. Though it is unlikely to occur with corticosteroids applied to the skin, this medication may affect growth in children if used for long periods. Monitor your child's height and rate of growth from time to time.

During pregnancy, this medication should be used only when clearly needed. Discuss the risks and benefits with your doctor.

It is not known whether this drug passes into breast milk when applied to the skin. Similar medications pass into breast milk when taken by mouth. Consult your doctor before breast-feeding.

Micatin

Micatin, an antifungal agent, is used for skin infections such as athlete's foot and jock itch and for vaginal yeast infections.

Micatin is a brand name for the generic drug Miconazole.

Micatin vaginal cream and suppositories are for use only in the vagina. These products are not to be taken by mouth. The vaginal suppositories are inserted, one per dose, in an applicator. Alternatively, the tube containing the vaginal cream is screwed onto the end of a special applicator tube, and the tube is then squeezed to fill the applicator. The patient then lies on her back with bent knees, inserts the applicator containing either the suppository or cream so that the tip of the applicator is high in the vagina, and then pushes the plunger in to deposit the suppository or cream into the vagina. The applicator should be washed with warm soap and water after each use.

Micatin usually is used once daily at bedtime. The 200 mg suppositories (Monistat 3) are inserted once nightly for 3 nights. The 100 mg suppositories

(Monistat-7) and intravaginal cream are inserted once nightly for 7 nights. The 1200 mg formulation (Monistat 1) is applied once for one night.

For fungal skin infections, the topical cream is applied as a thin layer to cover the affected skin and surrounding area, usually twice daily. The hands should be washed before and after application.

Micatin may cause the following side effects:
- Rash
- Burning at the site of application
- Itching
- Irritation of the skin or vagina
- Stomach pain
- Fever
- Foul-smelling vaginal discharge
- Diarrhea
- Vomiting
- Loss of appetite
- Hives
- Chills

There is very limited information on the use of Micatin during pregnancy. The physician must weigh the potential benefits against possible but unknown risks to the fetus.

It is not known if Micatin is secreted in breast milk in amounts that can affect the infant.

Tell your doctor about all the medicines you use (both prescription and nonprescription). Inform your doctor if you are taking:

- Anticoagulants (such as warfarin)
- Diabetes drugs
- Isoniazid
- Rifampin
- Rifabutin
- Phenytoin
- Cisapride

MICONAZOLE

Miconazole, an antifungal agent, is used for skin infections such as athlete's foot and jock itch and for vaginal yeast infections.

Miconazole is a generic drug sold under the brand names Desinex, Femizol, Fungoid, Lotrimin, Micatin, Monastat, Ting, Zeasorb, and possible others.

Miconazole vaginal cream and suppositories are for use only in the vagina. These products are not to be taken by mouth. The vaginal suppositories are inserted, one per dose, in an applicator. Alternatively, the tube containing the vaginal cream is screwed onto the end of a special applicator tube, and the tube is then squeezed to fill the applicator. The patient then lies on her back with bent knees, inserts the applicator containing either the suppository or cream so that the tip of the applicator is high in the vagina, and then pushes the plunger in to deposit the suppository or cream into the vagina. The applicator should be washed with warm soap and water after each use.

Miconazole usually is used once daily at bedtime. The 200 mg suppositories (Monistat 3) are inserted once nightly for 3 nights. The 100 mg suppositories (Monistat-7) and intravaginal cream are inserted once nightly for 7 nights. The 1200 mg formulation (Monistat 1) is applied once for one night.

For fungal skin infections, the topical cream is applied as a thin layer to cover the affected skin and surrounding area, usually twice daily. The hands should be washed before and after application.

Miconazole may cause the following side effects:

- Rash
- Burning at the site of application
- Itching
- Irritation of the skin or vagina
- Stomach pain
- Fever
- Foul-smelling vaginal discharge
- Diarrhea
- Vomiting
- Loss of appetite
- Hives
- Chills

There is very limited information on the use of miconazole during pregnancy. The physician must weigh the potential benefits against possible but unknown risks to the fetus.

It is not known if miconazole is secreted in breast milk in amounts that can affect the infant.

Tell your doctor about all the medicines you use (both prescription and nonprescription). Inform your doctor if you are taking:

- Anticoagulants (such as warfarin)
- Diabetes drugs
- Isoniazid
- Rifampin
- Rifabutin
- Phenytoin
- Cisapride

Monistat

Monistat, an antifungal agent, is used for skin infections such as athlete's foot and jock itch and for vaginal yeast infections.

Monistat is a brand name for the generic drug Miconazole.

Monistat vaginal cream and suppositories are for use only in the vagina. These products are not to be taken by mouth. The vaginal suppositories are inserted, one per dose, in an applicator. Alternatively, the tube containing the vaginal cream is screwed onto the end of a special applicator tube, and the tube is then squeezed to fill the applicator. The patient then lies on her back with bent knees, inserts the applicator containing either the suppository or cream so that the tip of the applicator is high in the vagina, and then pushes the plunger in to deposit the suppository or cream into the vagina. The applicator should be washed with warm soap and water after each use.

Monistat usually is used once daily at bedtime. The 200 mg suppositories (Monistat 3) are inserted once nightly for 3 nights. The 100 mg suppositories

(Monistat-7) and intravaginal cream are inserted once nightly for 7 nights. The 1200 mg formulation (Monistat 1) is applied once for one night.

For fungal skin infections, the topical cream is applied as a thin layer to cover the affected skin and surrounding area, usually twice daily. The hands should be washed before and after application.

Monistat may cause the following side effects:

- Rash
- Burning at the site of application
- Itching
- Irritation of the skin or vagina
- Stomach pain
- Fever
- Foul-smelling vaginal discharge
- Diarrhea
- Vomiting
- Loss of appetite
- Hives
- Chills

There is very limited information on the use of Monistat during pregnancy. The physician must weigh the potential benefits against possible but unknown risks to the fetus.

It is not known if Monistat is secreted in breast milk in amounts that can affect the infant.

Tell your doctor about all the medicines you use (both prescription and nonprescription). Inform your doctor if you are taking:

- Anticoagulants (such as warfarin)
- Diabetes drugs
- Isoniazid
- Rifampin
- Rifabutin
- Phenytoin
- Cisapride

Mycelex

Mycelex is prescribed to treat yeast infections of the vagina, mouth, and skin such as athlete's foot, jock itch, and body ringworm. It can also be used to prevent oral thrush in certain patients.

Mycelex is a brand name for the **drug** Clotrimazole.

Mycelex may cause the following **side effects:**

- Itching
- Burning
- Irritation
- Redness
- Swelling
- Stomach pain
- Fever
- Foul-smelling discharge if using the vaginal product
- Upset stomach or vomiting with the lozenges (troches)
- Extreme hair growth
- Skin thinning
- Skin discoloration
- Severe dizziness
- Trouble breathing
- Acne
- Stretch marks
- Hair bumps (folliculitis)

- ☠ Vision problems
- ☠ Persistent headache
- ☠ Increased thirst/urination
- ☠ Unusual weakness
- ☠ Sudden weight loss

Before using this medication, tell your doctor or pharmacist if you are allergic to clotrimazole or betamethasone; or to other azole antifungals (e.g., ketoconazole) or corticosteroids (e.g., triamcinolone); or if you have any other allergies.

Before using this medication, tell your doctor or pharmacist your medical history, especially of: immune system problems, poor blood circulation.

It is possible this medication will be absorbed into your bloodstream. This may have undesirable effects that may require additional corticosteroid treatment. Children and those using this drug for an extended time over most of the skin may be at higher risk, especially if they also have serious medical problems such as severe infections, injuries, or surgeries. This precaution applies for up to 1 year after stopping use of this drug.

Consult your doctor or pharmacist for more details, and tell them that you use (or have used) this medication.

Caution is advised when using this drug in the elderly because they may be more sensitive to the effects of the drug, especially thinning skin.

Caution is advised when using this drug in children because they may be more sensitive to the effects of too much steroid hormone. Though it is unlikely to occur with corticosteroids applied to the skin, this medication may affect growth in children if used for long periods. Monitor your child's height and rate of growth from time to time.

During pregnancy, this medication should be used only when clearly needed. Discuss the risks and benefits with your doctor.

It is not known whether this drug passes into breast milk when applied to the skin. Similar medications pass into breast milk when taken by mouth. Consult your doctor before breast-feeding.

Mycostatin

Mycostatin is prescribed to treat fungal infections of the skin, mouth, vagina, and intestinal tract.

Mycostatin is a brand name for the generic drug Nystatin.

Use of Mycostatin may cause the following side effects:

- Itching
- Irritation
- Burning
- Diarrhea
- Upset stomach
- Stomach pain
- Cramps
- Skin rash
- Nausea
- Vomiting
- Swelling
- Severe dizziness
- Trouble breathing

This medication should be used only when clearly needed during pregnancy. Discuss the risks and benefits with your doctor.

It is not known whether this drug passes into breast milk. Consult your doctor before breast-feeding.

Myco-Triacet

Myco-Triacet is prescribed to treat fungal infections of the skin, mouth, vagina, and intestinal tract.

Myco-Triacet is a brand name for the generic drug Nystatin.

Use of Myco-Triacet may cause the following side effects:

- Itching
- Irritation
- Burning
- Diarrhea
- Upset stomach
- Stomach pain
- Cramps
- Skin rash
- Nausea
- Vomiting
- Swelling
- Severe dizziness
- Trouble breathing

This medication should be used only when clearly needed during pregnancy. Discuss the risks and benefits with your doctor.

It is not known whether this drug passes into breast milk. Consult your doctor before breast-feeding.

Mytrex

Mytrex is prescribed to treat fungal infections of the skin, mouth, vagina, and intestinal tract.

Mytrex is a brand name for the generic drug Nystatin.

Use of Mytrex may cause the following side effects:

- Itching
- Irritation
- Burning
- Diarrhea
- Upset stomach
- Stomach pain
- Cramps
- Skin rash
- Nausea
- Vomiting
- Swelling
- Severe dizziness
- Trouble breathing

This medication should be used only when clearly needed during pregnancy. Discuss the risks and benefits with your doctor.

It is not known whether this drug passes into breast milk. Consult your doctor before breast-feeding.

Nizoral

Nizoral is prescribed to treat fungal infections. Nizoral is most often used to treat fungal infections that can spread to different parts of the body through the bloodstream such as yeast infections of the mouth, skin, urinary tract, and blood, and certain fungal infections that begin on the skin or in the lungs and can spread through the body. Nizoral is also used to treat fungal infections of the skin or nails that cannot be treated with other medications. Nizoral is in a class of antifungals called imidazoles. It works by slowing the growth of fungi that cause infection.

Nizoral is a brand name for the drug Ketoconazole.

Use of Nizoral has been associated with the following:

- Hepatotoxicity
- Headache
- Dizziness
- Tremors
- Nervousness
- Rash
- Swelling of the breasts
- Diarrhea

- ☠ Rectal bleeding
- ☠ Anemia
- ☠ Shock
- ☠ Cataract enlargement
- ☠ Shortness of breath
- ☠ Nausea
- ☠ Vomiting
- ☠ Abdominal pain
- ☠ Heartburn
- ☠ Extreme tiredness
- ☠ Loss of appetite
- ☠ Yellowing of skin or eyes
- ☠ Dark yellow urine
- ☠ Pale stools
- ☠ Pain in upper right part of stomach
- ☠ Flu-like symptoms

Nizoral may cause liver damage and should not be taken with:

- Acetaminophen (Tylenol, others)
- Cholesterol-lowering medications (statins) such as atorvastatin (Lipitor), fluvastatin (Lescol), lovastatin (Mevacor), pravastatin (Pravachol), or simvastatin (Zocor)
- Isoniazid (INH, Nydrazid)
- Methotrexate (Rheumatrex)
- Niacin (nicotinic acid)
- Rifampin
- Astemizole (Hismanal)

- Cisapride (Propulsid)
- Terfenadine (Seldane)

Tell your doctor and pharmacist what other prescription and nonprescription medications, vitamins, nutritional supplements, and herbal products you are taking any of the following:

- Alprazolam (Xanax)
- Anticoagulants ('blood thinners') such as warfarin (Coumadin)
- Buspirone (Buspar)
- Calcium channel blockers such as amlodipine (Norvasc), diltiazem (Cardizem, Dilacor, Tiazac), felodipine (Plendil), nifedipine (Adalat, Procardia), nisoldipine (Sular), and verapamil (Calan, Covera, Isoptin, Verelan)
- Clarithromycin (Biaxin)
- Cyclosporine (Neoral, Sandimmune)
- Diazepam (Valium)
- Digoxin (Lanoxin)
- Erythromycin (E.E.S., E-Mycin, Erythrocin)
- HIV protease inhibitors such as indinavir (Crixivan), ritonavir (Norvir), and

- saquinavir (Invirase, Fortovase)
- Loratadine (Claritin)
- Medications for diabetes
- Medications for erectile dysfunction such as sildenafil (Viagra), tadalafil (Cialis) and vardenafil (Levitra)
- Methadone (Dolophine)
- Methylprednisolone (Medrol)
- Midazolam (Versed)
- Phenytoin (Dilantin)
- Pimozide (Orap)
- Quinidine (Quinidex, Quinaglute)
- Quinine
- Tacrolimus (Prograf)
- Tamoxifen (Nolvadex)
- Telithromycin (Ketek)
- Trazodone (Desyrel)
- Vincristine (Vincasar)

Your doctor may need to change the doses of your medications or monitor you carefully for side effects.

if you are taking antacids; antihistamines; medications for heartburn or ulcers such as cimetidine (Tagamet), famotidine (Pepcid), nizatadine (Axid), or ranitidine (Zantac); or medications for irritable bowel disease, motion sickness, Parkinson's disease, ulcers, or urinary problems, take them 2 hours after you take Nizoral.

Tell your doctor if you are pregnant, plan to become pregnant, or are breast-feeding. If you become pregnant while taking Nizoral, call your doctor. Do not breastfeed while you are taking Nizoral.

Ask your doctor about the safe use of alcoholic beverages while you are taking Nizoral. You may experience unpleasant symptoms such as flushing, rash, upset stomach, headache, and swelling of the hands, feet, ankles, or lower legs if you drink alcohol while you are taking Nizoral.

Keep all appointments with your doctor and the laboratory. Your doctor will order certain tests to check your body's response to Nizoral.

Noxafil

Noxafil is an antifungal antibiotic that fights certain infections cause by fungus. Noxafil is used to prevent fungal infections in people with weak immune systems resulting from chemotherapy or stem cell transplantation. Noxafil is the brand name for the generic drug Posaconazole. It is available by prescription only.

Antibiotic medicines such as Noxafil can cause diarrhea, which may be a sign of a new infection. If you have diarrhea that is watery or has blood in it, call your doctor. Do not use any medicine to stop the diarrhea unless your doctor has told you to.

People who use Noxafil may experience some or all of these side effects:

- Easy bruising or bleeding
- Unusual weakness
- Fever
- Chills
- Cough
- Body aches
- Flu symptoms
- Fast heart rate
- Feeling light-headed

- ☠ Fainting
- ☠ Dry mouth
- ☠ Increased thirst
- ☠ Drowsiness
- ☠ Restless feeling
- ☠ Confusion
- ☠ Nausea
- ☠ Vomiting
- ☠ Increased urination
- ☠ Muscle pain or weakness
- ☠ Seizure (convulsions)
- ☠ Increased blood pressure
- ☠ Severe headache
- ☠ Blurred vision
- ☠ Trouble concentrating
- ☠ Chest pain
- ☠ Numbness
- ☠ Swelling of your ankles or feet
- ☠ White patches or sores inside your mouth or on your lips
- ☠ Nausea
- ☠ Stomach pain
- ☠ Low fever
- ☠ Loss of appetite
- ☠ Dark urine
- ☠ Clay-colored stools
- ☠ Jaundice (yellowing of the skin or eyes)
- ☠ Diarrhea that is watery or bloody
- ☠ Tired feeling
- ☠ Joint or muscle pain
- ☠ Sleep problems (insomnia)
- ☠ Dizziness
- ☠ Constipation

- ☠ Stomach pain
- ☠ Skin rash

Before taking Noxafil, tell your doctor if you are using any of the following drugs:

- Cimetidine (Tagamet)
- Cyclosporine (Neoral, Sandimmune, Gengraf)
- Midazolam (Versed)
- Phenytoin (Dilantin)
- Rifabutin (Mycobutin)
- Sirolimus (Rapamune)
- Tacrolimus (Prograf)
- Cancer medicines such as vinblastine (Velban) or vincristine (Oncovin, Vincasar), vindesine (Eldisine), or vinorelbine (Navelbine);
- Calcium channel blockers such as amlodipine (Norvasc), diltiazem (Tiazac, Cartia, Cardizem), felodipine (Plendil), nicardipine (Cardene), nifedipine (Procardia, Adalat), nimodipine (Nimotop), nisoldipine (Sular), or verapamil (Calan, Covera, Isoptin, Verelan)
- Cholesterol-lowering medicines such as lovastatin (Mevacor), simvastatin

(Zocor), pravastatin (Pravachol), fluvastatin (Lescol), atorvastatin (Lipitor), or cerivastatin (Baycol)

If you are using any of these drugs, you may not be able to use Noxafil, or you may need dosage adjustments or special tests during treatment.

There may be other drugs not listed that can affect Noxafil. Tell your doctor about all the prescription and over-the-counter medications you use. This includes vitamins, minerals, herbal products, and drugs prescribed by other doctors. Do not start using a new medication without telling your doctor.

You should not take Noxafil if you are using any of the following drugs:

- Astemizole (Hismanal)
- Cisapride (Propulsid)
- Halofantrine (Halfan)
- Pimozide (Orap)
- Quinidine (Cardioquin, Quinidex, Quinaglute)
- Terfenadine (Seldane)
- Methysergide (Sansert)
- Ergotamine (Ergomar, Ergostat, Cafergot, Ercaf, Wigraine)

- Dihydroergotamine (D.H.E. 45, Migranal Nasal Spray)
- Ergonovine (Ergotrate)
- Methylergonovine (Methergine)

Noxafil may be harmful to an unborn baby. Tell your doctor if you are pregnant or plan to become pregnant during treatment. It is not known whether Noxafil passes into breast milk or if it could harm a nursing baby. Do not use this medication without telling your doctor if you are breast-feeding a baby.

Do not Noxafil to a child younger than 13 years old.

To be sure Noxafil is not causing harmful effects your blood will need to be tested on a regular basis. Your liver function may also need to be tested. Do not miss any scheduled visits to your doctor.

It is very important to take the exact amount prescribed. Shake the oral suspension (liquid) well just before you measure a dose. To be sure you get the correct dose, measure the liquid with a marked measuring spoon or medicine cup, not with a regular table spoon. If you do not have a dose-measuring device, ask your pharmacist for one.   Do not take this medication without an exact measurement of the amount you are taking.

Nystat

Nystat is prescribed to treat fungal infections of the skin, mouth, vagina, and intestinal tract.

Nystat is a brand name for the generic drug Nystatin.

Use of Nystat may cause the following side effects:

- Itching
- Irritation
- Burning
- Diarrhea
- Upset stomach
- Stomach pain
- Cramps
- Skin rash
- Nausea
- Vomiting
- Swelling
- Severe dizziness
- Trouble breathing

This medication should be used only when clearly needed during pregnancy. Discuss the risks and benefits with your doctor.

It is not known whether this drug passes into breast milk. Consult your doctor before breast-feeding.

Nystatin

Nystatin is prescribed to treat fungal infections of the skin, mouth, vagina, and intestinal tract.

Nystatin is a generic drug sold under the brand names Myco-Triacet, Mytrex, Mycostatin, Nystat, Nystop, and possibly others.

Use of Nystatin may cause the following side effects:

- Itching
- Irritation
- Burning
- Diarrhea
- Upset stomach
- Stomach pain
- Cramps
- Skin rash
- Nausea
- Vomiting
- Swelling
- Severe dizziness
- Trouble breathing

This medication should be used only when clearly needed during pregnancy. Discuss the risks and benefits with your doctor.

It is not known whether this drug passes into breast milk. Consult your doctor before breast-feeding.

Nystop

Nystop is prescribed to treat fungal infections of the skin, mouth, vagina, and intestinal tract.

Nystop is a brand name for the generic drug Nystatin.

Use of Nystop may cause the following side effects:

- Itching
- Irritation
- Burning
- Diarrhea
- Upset stomach
- Stomach pain
- Cramps
- Skin rash
- Nausea
- Vomiting
- Swelling
- Severe dizziness
- Trouble breathing

This medication should be used only when clearly needed during pregnancy. Discuss the risks and benefits with your doctor.

It is not known whether this drug passes into breast milk. Consult your doctor before breast-feeding.

Posaconazole

Posaconazole is an antifungal antibiotic that fights certain infections cause by fungus. Posaconazole is used to prevent fungal infections in people with weak immune systems resulting from chemotherapy or stem cell transplantation. Posaconazole is the generic name for the brand name drug Noxafil. It is available by prescription only.

Antibiotic medicines such as Posaconazole can cause diarrhea, which may be a sign of a new infection. If you have diarrhea that is watery or has blood in it, call your doctor. Do not use any medicine to stop the diarrhea unless your doctor has told you to.

People who use Posaconazole may experience some or all of these side effects:

- Easy bruising or bleeding
- Unusual weakness
- Fever
- Chills
- Cough
- Body aches
- Flu symptoms

- ☠ Fast heart rate
- ☠ Feeling light-headed
- ☠ Fainting
- ☠ Dry mouth
- ☠ Increased thirst
- ☠ Drowsiness
- ☠ Restless feeling
- ☠ Confusion
- ☠ Nausea
- ☠ Vomiting
- ☠ Increased urination
- ☠ Muscle pain or weakness
- ☠ Seizure (convulsions)
- ☠ Increased blood pressure
- ☠ Severe headache
- ☠ Blurred vision
- ☠ Trouble concentrating
- ☠ Chest pain
- ☠ Numbness
- ☠ Swelling of your ankles or feet
- ☠ White patches or sores inside your mouth or on your lips
- ☠ Nausea
- ☠ Stomach pain
- ☠ Low fever
- ☠ Loss of appetite
- ☠ Dark urine
- ☠ Clay-colored stools
- ☠ Jaundice (yellowing of the skin or eyes)
- ☠ Diarrhea that is watery or bloody
- ☠ Tired feeling
- ☠ Joint or muscle pain
- ☠ Sleep problems (insomnia)

- ☠ Dizziness
- ☠ Constipation
- ☠ Stomach pain
- ☠ Skin rash

Before taking Posaconazole, tell your doctor if you are using any of the following drugs:

- Cimetidine (Tagamet)
- Cyclosporine (Neoral, Sandimmune, Gengraf)
- Midazolam (Versed)
- Phenytoin (Dilantin)
- Rifabutin (Mycobutin)
- Sirolimus (Rapamune)
- Tacrolimus (Prograf)
- Cancer medicines such as vinblastine (Velban) or vincristine (Oncovin, Vincasar), vindesine (Eldisine), or vinorelbine (Navelbine);
- Calcium channel blockers such as amlodipine (Norvasc), diltiazem (Tiazac, Cartia, Cardizem), felodipine (Plendil), nicardipine (Cardene), nifedipine (Procardia, Adalat), nimodipine (Nimotop), nisoldipine (Sular), or

> verapamil (Calan, Covera, Isoptin, Verelan)
- Cholesterol-lowering medicines such as lovastatin (Mevacor), simvastatin (Zocor), pravastatin (Pravachol), fluvastatin (Lescol), atorvastatin (Lipitor), or cerivastatin (Baycol)

If you are using any of these drugs, you may not be able to use Posaconazole, or you may need dosage adjustments or special tests during treatment.

There may be other drugs not listed that can affect Posaconazole. Tell your doctor about all the prescription and over-the-counter medications you use. This includes vitamins, minerals, herbal products, and drugs prescribed by other doctors. Do not start using a new medication without telling your doctor.

You should not take Posaconazole if you are using any of the following drugs:

- Astemizole (Hismanal)
- Cisapride (Propulsid)
- Halofantrine (Halfan)
- Pimozide (Orap)

- Quinidine (Cardioquin, Quinidex, Quinaglute)
- Terfenadine (Seldane)
- Methysergide (Sansert)
- Ergotamine (Ergomar, Ergostat, Cafergot, Ercaf, Wigraine)
- Dihydroergotamine (D.H.E. 45, Migranal Nasal Spray)
- Ergonovine (Ergotrate)
- Methylergonovine (Methergine)

Posaconazole may be harmful to an unborn baby. Tell your doctor if you are pregnant or plan to become pregnant during treatment. It is not known whether posaconazole passes into breast milk or if it could harm a nursing baby. Do not use this medication without telling your doctor if you are breast-feeding a baby.

Do not give Posaconazole to a child younger than 13 years old.

To be sure Posaconazole is not causing harmful effects your blood will need to be tested on a regular basis. Your liver function may also need to be tested. Do not miss any scheduled visits to your doctor.

It is very important to take the exact amount prescribed. Shake the oral suspension (liquid) well just before you measure a dose. To be sure you get the correct dose, measure the liquid with a marked measuring spoon or medicine cup, not with a regular table spoon. If you do not have a dose-measuring device, ask your pharmacist for one. Do not take this medication without an exact measurement of the amount you are taking.

Sporanox

Sporanox capsules are prescribed to treat fungal infections that begin in the lungs and can spread through the body. Sporanox capsules are also used to treat fungal infections of the fingernails and/or toenails. Sporanox oral solution is used to treat yeast infections of the mouth and throat and suspected fungal infections in patients with fever and certain other signs of infection. Sporanox is in a class of antifungals called triazoles. It works by slowing the growth of fungi that cause infection.

Sporanox is a brand name for the drug Itraconazole.

Sporanox can cause congestive heart failure (condition in which the heart cannot pump enough blood through the body).

Tell your doctor if you have or have ever had heart failure; a heart attack; an irregular heartbeat; any other type of heart disease; lung, liver, or kidney disease; or any other serious health problem.

If you experience any of the following symptoms, stop taking Sporanox and, call your doctor immediately:

- ☠ Shortness of breath
- ☠ Coughing up white or pink phlegm
- ☠ Weakness
- ☠ Excessive tiredness
- ☠ Fast heartbeat
- ☠ Swelling of the feet, ankles, or legs
- ☠ Sudden weight gain
- ☠ People who take Sporanox may experience the following side effects:
- ☠ Diarrhea or loose stools
- ☠ Constipation
- ☠ Gas
- ☠ Stomach pain
- ☠ Heartburn
- ☠ Sore or bleeding gums
- ☠ Sores in or around the mouth
- ☠ Headache
- ☠ Dizziness
- ☠ Sweating
- ☠ Muscle pain
- ☠ Decreased sexual desire or ability
- ☠ Nervousness
- ☠ Depression
- ☠ Runny nose and other cold symptoms
- ☠ Unusual dreams
- ☠ Excessive tiredness
- ☠ Loss of appetite
- ☠ Upset stomach

- ☠ Vomiting
- ☠ Yellowing of the skin or eyes
- ☠ Dark urine
- ☠ Pale stools
- ☠ Tingling or numbness of the hands or feet
- ☠ Fever, chills, or other signs of infection
- ☠ Frequent or painful urination
- ☠ Shaking hands that you cannot control
- ☠ Rash
- ☠ Hives
- ☠ Itching
- ☠ Difficulty breathing or swallowing

Use of Sporanox has been associated with serious hepatotoxicity, including liver failure and death. Some of these cases occurred within the first week of use.

Life-threatening irregularities in heart rhythms (cardiac dysrhythmias), and sudden death have occurred when patients were using medications in addition to Sporanox, such as Quinidine. Cases of congestive heart failure and pulmonary edema have also been experienced.

Do not take the following medications while you are taking Sporanox. If you do you may experience serious irregular heartbeats:

- Cisapride (Propulsid)
- Dofetilide (Tikosyn)
- Pimozide (Orap)
- Quinidine (Quinaglute, Quinidex, others)

Talk to your doctor about the risks of taking Sporanox.

Tell your doctor and pharmacist if you are allergic to Sporanox; other antifungal medications such as fluconazole (Diflucan), ketoconazole (Nizoral), or voriconazole (Vfend); or any other medications.

If you are taking Sporanox oral solution, tell your doctor if you are allergic to saccharin or sulfa medications.

Do not take Sporanox if you are taking any of the following medications:

- Ergot-type medications such as dihydroergotamine (D.H.E. 45, Migranal)
- Ergoloid mesylates (Germinal, Hydergine)
- Ergonovine (Ergotrate)
- Ergotamine (Bellergal-S, Cafergot, Ergomar, Wigraine)

- Methylergonovine (Methergine)
- Methysergide (Sansert)
- Lovastatin (Mevacor)
- Simvastatin (Zocor)
- Triazolam (Halcion)

Tell your doctor and pharmacist what other prescription and nonprescription medications, vitamins, nutritional supplements and herbal products you are taking, especially:

- Alfentanil (Alfenta)
- Alprazolam (Xanax)
- Anticoagulants (blood thinners) such as warfarin (Coumadin)
- Atorvastatin (Lipitor)
- Buspirone (BuSpar)
- Busulfan (Myleran)
- Calcium channel blockers such as amlodipine (Norvasc), felodipine (Plendil), isradipine (Dynacirc), nifedipine (Adalat, Procardia) nicardipine (Cardene) nimodipine (Nimotop), nisoldipine (Sular), and verapamil (Calan, Covera, Isoptin, Verelan)
- Carbamazepine (Tegretol)

- Cerivastatin (Baycol) (not available in the United States)
- Cilostazol (Pletal)
- Clarithromycin (Biaxin)
- Cyclosporine (Neoral, Sandimmune)
- Diazepam (Valium)
- Digoxin (Lanoxin)
- Disopyramide (Norpace)
- Docetaxel (Taxotere)
- Eletriptan (Relpax)
- Erythromycin (E.E.S., Erythrocin, E-Mycin)
- Halofantrine (Halfan)
- HIV protease inhibitors such as indinavir (Crixivan), ritonavir (Norvir), and saquinavir (Fortovase, Invirase)
- Isoniazid (INH, Nydrazid)
- Medications for erectile dysfunction such as sildenafil (Viagra), tadalafil (Cialis), and vardenafil (Levitra)
- Midazolam (Versed)
- Nevirapine (Viramune)
- Oral contraceptives (birth control pills)
- Oral medicine for diabetes
- Phenobarbital (Luminal, Solfoton)
- Phenytoin (Dilantin)
- Rifabutin (Mycobutin)

- Rifampin (Rifadin, Rimactane)
- Sirolimus (Rapamune)
- Steroids such as dexamethasone (Decadron), budesonide (Entocort EC), and methylprednisolone (Medrol)
- Tacrolimus (Prograf)
- Trimetrexate (Neutrexin)
- Vinblastine (Velban)
- Vincristine (Oncovin)
- Vinorelbine (Navelbine)

Many other medications may also interact with Sporanox, so be sure to tell your doctor about all the medications you are taking, even those that do not appear on this list.

You should know that Sporanox may remain in your body for several months after you stop taking it. Tell your doctor that you have recently stopped taking Sporanox before you start taking any other medications during the first few months after your treatment.

If you are taking an antacid, take it 1 hour before or 2 hours after you take Sporanox.
Tell your doctor if you have or have ever had AIDS, cystic fibrosis (an inborn disease that causes problems with

breathing, digestion, and reproduction), or any condition that decreases the amount of acid in your stomach.

Tell your doctor if you are pregnant, plan to become pregnant, or are breast-feeding. You should not take Sporanox to treat nail fungus if you are pregnant or could become pregnant. You may start to take Sporanox to treat nail fungus only on the second or third day of your menstrual period when you are sure you are not pregnant. You must use effective birth control during your treatment and for 2 months afterward. If you become pregnant while taking Sporanox to treat any condition, call your doctor immediately.

One of the ingredients in Sporanox oral solution caused cancer in some types of laboratory animals. It is not known whether people who take Sporanox solution have an increased risk of developing cancer. Talk to your doctor about the risks of taking Sporanox solution.

Terazol

Terazol is used to treat fungal and yeast infections of the vagina. Terazol comes as a cream and suppository to insert into the vagina. It is usually used daily at bedtime for either 3 or 7 days. Always follow the directions on your prescription label carefully, and ask your doctor or pharmacist to explain any part you do not understand. Use Terazol exactly as directed. Do not use more or less of it or use it more often than prescribed by your doctor.

Terazol a brand name for the drug Terconazole.

Terazol may cause these side effects:

- Headache
- Missed menstrual periods
- Burning in vagina
- Irritation in vagina
- Stomach pain
- Fever
- Chills
- Flu-like symptoms
- Foul-smelling vaginal discharge

Terazol is for external use only. Do not let cream get into your eyes or mouth, and do not swallow it.

Refrain from sexual intercourse. An ingredient in the cream may weaken certain latex products like condoms or diaphragms; do not use such products within 72 hours of using this medication. Wear clean cotton panties (or panties with cotton crotches), not panties made of nylon, rayon, or other synthetic fabrics.

It is not known whether this drug is excreted in human milk. Animal studies have shown that offspring exposed via mother's milk of showed decreased survival during the first few post-partum days. Because many drugs are excreted in human milk, and because of the potential for adverse reaction in nursing infants from Terazol, a decision should be made whether to discontinue nursing or to discontinue the drug, taking into account the importance of the drug to the mother.

TERBINAFINE

Terbinafine is used to treat fungal infections of the toenail and fingernail. Terbinafine is in a class of medications called antifungals. It works by stopping the growth of fungi. Terbinafine comes as a tablet to take by mouth. It is usually taken once a day for 6 weeks for fingernail fungus and once a day for 12 weeks for toenail fungus. Follow the directions on your prescription label carefully, and ask your doctor or pharmacist to explain any part you do not understand. Take Terbinafine exactly as directed. Do not take more or less of it or take it more often than prescribed by your doctor.

Terbinafine is a generic drug sold under the brand name Lamisil.

Use of Terbinafine has been associated with the following:

- ☠ Liver failure, leading to liver transplant or death
- ☠ Serious skin reactions
- ☠ Serious blood disorders
- ☠ Rash
- ☠ Eczema
- ☠ Itch

- ☠ Diarrhea
- ☠ Abdominal pain
- ☠ Nausea
- ☠ Vomiting
- ☠ Headache
- ☠ Fatigue
- ☠ Muscle and joint pain
- ☠ Hypoglycemia
- ☠ Change in taste or loss of taste
- ☠ Hives
- ☠ Loss of appetite
- ☠ Vomiting
- ☠ Extreme tiredness
- ☠ Pain in the right upper part of stomach
- ☠ Dark urine
- ☠ Pale stools
- ☠ Fever
- ☠ Sore throat

Tell your doctor and pharmacist what prescription and nonprescription medications, vitamins, nutritional supplements, and herbal products you are taking.

Be sure to mention any of the following:

- Anticoagulants (blood thinners) such as warfarin (Coumadin)
- Antidepressants such as amitriptyline (Elavil), amoxapine (Asendin),

- clomipramine (Anafranil), desipramine (Norpramin), doxepin (Adapin, Sinequan), imipramine (Tofranil), nortriptyline (Aventyl, Pamelor), protriptyline (Vivactil), and trimipramine (Surmontil)
- Beta-blockers such as atenolol (Tenormin), labetalol (Normodyne), metoprolol (Lopressor, Toprol XL), nadolol (Corgard), and propranolol (Inderal)
- Cimetidine (Tagamet)
- Medications that suppress the immune system such as azathioprine (Imuran), cyclosporine (Neoral, Sandimmune), methotrexate (Rheumatrex), sirolimus (Rapamune), and tacrolimus (Prograf)
- Rifampin (Rifadin, Rimactane); and selegiline (Eldepryl)

If you use any of the above drugs your doctor may need to change the doses of your medications or monitor you carefully for side effects.

Tell your doctor if you have or have ever had kidney or liver disease, human immunodeficiency virus (HIV), or acquired immunodeficiency syndrome (AIDS).

Tell your doctor if you are pregnant, plan to become pregnant, or are breast-feeding. If you become pregnant while taking Terbinafine, call your doctor immediately. You should not take Terbinafine while breast-feeding.

Terconazole

Terconazole is used to treat fungal and yeast infections of the vagina. Terconazole comes as a cream and suppository to insert into the vagina. It is usually used daily at bedtime for either 3 or 7 days. Always follow the directions on your prescription label carefully, and ask your doctor or pharmacist to explain any part you do not understand. Use terconazole exactly as directed. Do not use more or less of it or use it more often than prescribed by your doctor.

Terconazole is available under the brand name Terazol.

Terconazole may cause these side effects:

- Headache
- Missed menstrual periods
- Burning in vagina
- Irritation in vagina
- Stomach pain
- Fever
- Chills
- Flu-like symptoms
- Foul-smelling vaginal discharge

Terconazole is for external use only. Do not let cream get into your eyes or mouth, and do not swallow it.

Refrain from sexual intercourse. An ingredient in the cream may weaken certain latex products like condoms or diaphragms; do not use such products within 72 hours of using this medication. Wear clean cotton panties (or panties with cotton crotches), not panties made of nylon, rayon, or other synthetic fabrics.

It is not known whether this drug is excreted in human milk. Animal studies have shown that offspring exposed via mother's milk of showed decreased survival during the first few post-partum days. Because many drugs are excreted in human milk, and because of the potential for adverse reaction in nursing infants from Terconazole, a decision should be made whether to discontinue nursing or to discontinue the drug, taking into account the importance of the drug to the mother.

Tinidazole

Tinidazole is used to treat trichomoniasis (a sexually transmitted disease that can affect men and women), giardiasis (an infection of the intestine that can cause diarrhea, gas, and stomach cramps), and amebiasis (an infection of the intestine that can cause diarrhea, gas, and stomach cramps and can spread to other organs such as the liver). Tinidazole is in a class of medications called antiprotozoal agents. It works by killing the organisms that can cause infection.

Tinidazole is a generic drug sold under the brand name Tindamax.

Tinidazole comes as a suspension (liquid) prepared by the pharmacist and a tablet to take by mouth. It is usually taken with food as a single dose or once a day for 3 to 5 days. To help you remember to take tinidazole (if you are to take it for more than one day), take it around the same time every day. Follow the directions on your prescription label carefully, and ask your doctor or pharmacist to explain any part you do not understand. Take tinidazole exactly as directed. Do not take more or less of it or take it more often than prescribed by your doctor.

Tell your doctor and pharmacist what prescription and nonprescription medications, vitamins, nutritional supplements, and herbal products you are taking. Be sure to mention any of the following:

- Anticoagulants (blood thinners) such as warfarin (Coumadin)
- Antifungals such as fluconazole (Diflucan), Sporanox (Sporanox), and ketoconazole (Nizoral)
- Carbamazepine (Tegretol)
- Cimetidine (Tagamet)
- Clarithromycin (Biaxin)
- Cyclosporine (Neoral, Sandimmune)
- Danazol (Danocrine)
- Delavirdine (Rescriptor)
- Dexamethasone (Decadron)
- Diltiazem (Cardizem, Dilacor; Tiazac)
- Erythromycin (E.E.S., E-Mycin, Erythrocin)
- Ethosuximide (Zarontin)
- Fluorouracil (Adrucil)
- Fluoxetine (Prozac, Sarafem)
- Fluvoxamine (Luvox)
- Fosphenytoin (Cerebyx)

- HIV protease inhibitors such as indinavir (Crixivan) and ritonavir (Norvir)
- Isoniazid (INH, Nydrazid)
- Lithium (Lithobid)
- Metronidazole (Flagyl)
- Nefazodone (Serzone)
- Oral contraceptives (birth control pills)
- Oxytetracycline (Terramycin)
- Phenobarbital (Luminal, Solfoton)
- Phenytoin (Dilantin)
- Rifabutin (Mycobutin)
- Rifampin (Rifadin, Rimactane)
- Tacrolimus (Prograf)
- Troglitazone (Rezulin)
- Troleandomycin (TAO)
- Verapamil (Calan, Covera, Isoptin, Verelan)
- Zafirlukast (Accolate).

Also tell your doctor if you are taking Disulfiram (Antabuse) or have stopped taking it within the past 2 weeks. Your doctor may need to change the doses of your medications or monitor you carefully for side effects.

If you are taking Cholestyramine (Questran), you should not take it at the same time that you take Tinidazole. Ask your doctor or pharmacist how to space doses of these medications.

Tell your doctor if you have a yeast infection now; if you are being treated with dialysis (mechanical removal of waste in patients with kidney failure); or if you have or have ever had seizures or nervous system, blood, or liver disease.

Know that you should not drink alcohol while you are taking this medication and for 3 days afterwards. Alcohol may cause an upset stomach, vomiting, stomach cramps, headaches, sweating, and flushing (redness of the face).

Talk to your doctor about drinking grapefruit juice while taking this medication.

Tinidazole is known to cause the following side effects. :

- Sharp, unpleasant metallic taste
- Upset stomach
- Vomiting
- Loss of appetite
- Constipation
- Stomach pain or cramps
- Headache
- Tiredness or weakness
- Dizziness
- Seizures

- ☠ Numbness or tingling of hands or feet
- ☠ Rash
- ☠ Hives
- ☠ Swelling of the face, throat, tongue, lips, eyes, hands, feet, ankles, or lower legs
- ☠ Hoarseness
- ☠ Difficulty swallowing or breathing

Keep all appointments with your doctor and the laboratory. Your doctor may order certain lab tests to check your body's response to Tinidazole. Before having any laboratory test, tell your doctor and the laboratory personnel that you are taking Tinidazole.

Another medication that is similar to Tinidazole has caused cancer in laboratory animals. It is not known whether Tinidazole increases the risk of developing cancer in laboratory animals or in humans. Talk to your doctor about the risks and benefits of using this medication.

Tell your doctor if you are pregnant or plan to become pregnant. If you become pregnant while taking Tinidazole, call your doctor immediately. The use of Tinidazole in pregnant patients has not been studied. Since Tinidazole crosses the placental barrier and enters fetal circulation it should not be administered to pregnant patients in the first trimester.

Tinidazole is excreted in breast milk in concentrations similar to those seen in serum. Tinidazole can be detected in breast milk for up to 72 hours following administration. Interruption of breast-feeding is recommended during tinidazole therapy and for 3 days following the last dose.

Tindamax

Tindamax is used to treat trichomoniasis (a sexually transmitted disease that can affect men and women), giardiasis (an infection of the intestine that can cause diarrhea, gas, and stomach cramps), and amebiasis (an infection of the intestine that can cause diarrhea, gas, and stomach cramps and can spread to other organs such as the liver). Tindamax is in a class of medications called antiprotozoal agents. It works by killing the organisms that can cause infection.

Tindamax is a brand name for the drug Tinidazole.

Tindamax comes as a suspension (liquid) prepared by the pharmacist and a tablet to take by mouth. It is usually taken with food as a single dose or once a day for 3 to 5 days. To help you remember to take Tindamax (if you are to take it for more than one day), take it around the same time every day. Follow the directions on your prescription label carefully, and ask your doctor or pharmacist to explain any part you do not understand. Take Tindamax exactly as directed. Do not take more or less of it or take it more often than prescribed by your doctor.

Tell your doctor and pharmacist what prescription and nonprescription medications, vitamins, nutritional supplements, and herbal products you are taking. Be sure to mention any of the following:

- Anticoagulants (blood thinners) such as warfarin (Coumadin)
- Antifungals such as fluconazole (Diflucan), itraconazole (Sporanox), and Ketoconazole (Nizoral)
- Carbamazepine (Tegretol)
- Cimetidine (Tagamet)
- Clarithromycin (Biaxin)
- Cyclosporine (Neoral, Sandimmune)
- Danazol (Danocrine)
- Delavirdine (Rescriptor)
- Dexamethasone (Decadron)
- Diltiazem (Cardizem, Dilacor; Tiazac)
- Erythromycin (E.E.S., E-Mycin, Erythrocin)
- Ethosuximide (Zarontin)
- Fluorouracil (Adrucil)
- Fluoxetine (Prozac, Sarafem)
- Fluvoxamine (Luvox)
- Fosphenytoin (Cerebyx)

- HIV protease inhibitors such as indinavir (Crixivan) and ritonavir (Norvir)
- Isoniazid (INH, Nydrazid)
- Lithium (Lithobid)
- Metronidazole (Flagyl)
- Nefazodone (Serzone)
- Oral contraceptives (birth control pills)
- Oxytetracycline (Terramycin)
- Phenobarbital (Luminal, Solfoton)
- Phenytoin (Dilantin)
- Rifabutin (Mycobutin)
- Rifampin (Rifadin, Rimactane)
- Tacrolimus (Prograf)
- Troglitazone (Rezulin)
- Troleandomycin (TAO)
- Verapamil (Calan, Covera, Isoptin, Verelan)
- Zafirlukast (Accolate)

Also tell your doctor if you are taking Disulfiram (Antabuse) or have stopped taking it within the past 2 weeks. Your doctor may need to change the doses of your medications or monitor you carefully for side effects.

If you are taking Cholestyramine (Questran), you should not take it at the same time that you take Tindamax. Ask your doctor or pharmacist how to space doses of these medications.

Tell your doctor if you have a yeast infection now; if you are being treated with dialysis (mechanical removal of waste in patients with kidney failure); or if you have or have ever had seizures or nervous system, blood, or liver disease.

Know that you should not drink alcohol while you are taking this medication and for 3 days afterwards. Alcohol may cause an upset stomach, vomiting, stomach cramps, headaches, sweating, and flushing (redness of the face).

Talk to your doctor about drinking grapefruit juice while taking this medication.

Tindamax is known to cause the following side effects. :

- Sharp, unpleasant metallic taste
- Upset stomach
- Vomiting
- Loss of appetite
- Constipation
- Stomach pain or cramps
- Headache
- Tiredness or weakness
- Dizziness
- Seizures

- ☠ Numbness or tingling of hands or feet
- ☠ Rash
- ☠ Hives
- ☠ Swelling of the face, throat, tongue, lips, eyes, hands, feet, ankles, or lower legs
- ☠ Hoarseness
- ☠ Difficulty swallowing or breathing

Keep all appointments with your doctor and the laboratory. Your doctor may order certain lab tests to check your body's response to Tindamax. Before having any laboratory test, tell your doctor and the laboratory personnel that you are taking Tindamax.

Another medication that is similar to Tindamax has caused cancer in laboratory animals. It is not known whether Tindamax increases the risk of developing cancer in laboratory animals or in humans. Talk to your doctor about the risks and benefits of using this medication.

Tell your doctor if you are pregnant or plan to become pregnant. If you become pregnant while taking Tindamax, call your doctor immediately. The use of Tindamax in pregnant patients has not been studied. Since Tindamax crosses the placental barrier and enters fetal circulation it should not be administered to pregnant patients in the first trimester.

Tindamax is excreted in breast milk in concentrations similar to those seen in serum. Tindamax can be detected in breast milk for up to 72 hours following administration. Interruption of breast-feeding is recommended during Tindamax therapy and for 3 days following the last dose.

Ting

Ting, an antifungal agent, is used for skin infections such as athlete's foot and jock itch and for vaginal yeast infections.

Ting is a brand name for the generic drug Miconazole.

Ting vaginal cream and suppositories are for use only in the vagina. These products are not to be taken by mouth. The vaginal suppositories are inserted, one per dose, in an applicator. Alternatively, the tube containing the vaginal cream is screwed onto the end of a special applicator tube, and the tube is then squeezed to fill the applicator. The patient then lies on her back with bent knees, inserts the applicator containing either the suppository or cream so that the tip of the applicator is high in the vagina, and then pushes the plunger in to deposit the suppository or cream into the vagina. The applicator should be washed with warm soap and water after each use.

Ting usually is used once daily at bedtime. The 200 mg suppositories (Monistat 3) are inserted once nightly for 3 nights. The 100 mg suppositories

(Monistat-7) and intravaginal cream are inserted once nightly for 7 nights. The 1200 mg formulation (Monistat 1) is applied once for one night.

For fungal skin infections, the topical cream is applied as a thin layer to cover the affected skin and surrounding area, usually twice daily. The hands should be washed before and after application.

Ting may cause the following side effects:

- Rash
- Burning at the site of application
- Itching
- Irritation of the skin or vagina
- Stomach pain
- Fever
- Foul-smelling vaginal discharge
- Diarrhea
- Vomiting
- Loss of appetite
- Hives
- Chills

There is very limited information on the use of Ting during pregnancy. The physician must weigh the potential benefits against possible but unknown risks to the fetus.

It is not known if Ting is secreted in breast milk in amounts that can affect the infant.

Tell your doctor about all the medicines you use (both prescription and nonprescription). Inform your doctor if you are taking:

- Anticoagulants (such as warfarin)
- Diabetes drugs
- Isoniazid
- Rifampin
- Rifabutin
- Phenytoin
- Cisapride

Tioconazole

Tioconazole is an antifungal medication. It prevents fungus from growing. It is used to treat vaginal Candida (yeast) infections.

Tioconazole is a generic drug sold under the brand named Vagistat.

Avoid using condoms, cervical caps, or vaginal contraceptive diaphragms for 3 days following treatment with Tioconazole. Tioconazole contains oils that can weaken latex rubber condoms, diaphragms, or cervical caps. This increases the chance of a condom breaking during sex. The rubber in a cervical cap or diaphragm can also break down faster and wear out sooner.

Vaginal medicines usually will come out of the vagina during treatment. To keep the medicine from getting on your clothing, wear a minipad or sanitary napkin. The use of tampons is not recommended since they may soak up the medicine. To help clear up the infection, wear freshly washed cotton, not synthetic, underwear.

Side effects experienced when taking Tioconazole may include:

- ☠ Shortness of breath
- ☠ Closing of your throat
- ☠ Swelling of your lips, face, or tongue
- ☠ Hives
- ☠ Burning
- ☠ Itching
- ☠ Irritation of the skin
- ☠ Increased need to urinate

Do not use Tioconazole if you have a fever, abdominal pain, foul-smelling discharge, diabetes, HIV, or AIDS.

This means that it is not known whether Tioconazole vaginal will be harmful to an unborn baby. Do not use this medication without first talking to your doctor if you are pregnant or could become pregnant during treatment.

It is not known whether Tioconazole passes into breast milk. Do not use Tioconazole vaginal without first talking to your doctor if you are breast-feeding a baby.

Trican

Trican is used to treat fungal infections, including yeast infections of the vagina, mouth, throat, esophagus (tube leading from the mouth to the stomach), abdomen (area between the chest and waist), lungs, blood, and other organs. Trican is also used to treat meningitis (infection of the membranes covering the brain and spine) caused by fungus. Trican is also used to prevent yeast infections in patients who are likely to become infected because they are being treated with chemotherapy or radiation therapy before a bone marrow transplant (replacement of unhealthy spongy tissue inside the bones with healthy tissue). Trican is in a class of antifungals called triazoles. It works by slowing the growth of fungi that cause infection.

Trican is a brand name for the drug Fluconazole.

Use of Trican has been associated with liver (hepatic) injury, including death, in patients with serious underlying medical conditions.

Cases of severe reaction leading to skin loss (exfoliative disorder) have been recorded.

Approximately 26% of patients experience some adverse side effects from Trican including:

- Headache
- Dizziness
- Diarrhea
- Stomach pain
- Heartburn
- Change in ability to taste food
- Mistaking one taste for another
- Upset stomach
- Extreme tiredness
- Unusual bruising or bleeding
- Lack of energy
- Loss of appetite
- Pain in the upper right part of the stomach
- Yellowing of the skin or eyes
- Flu-like symptoms
- Dark urine
- Pale stools
- Seizures
- Rash
- Hives
- Itching
- Swelling of the face, throat, tongue, lips, eyes, hands, feet, ankles, or lower legs
- Difficulty breathing

- ☠ Difficulty swallowing
- ☠ Indigestion
- ☠ Nausea

Trican therapy has been associated with QT interval prolongation, which may lead to serious cardiac arrhythmias. Thus it is used with caution in patients with risk factors for prolonged QT interval such as electrolyte imbalance or use of other drugs which may prolong the QT interval (particularly cisapride).
High concentrations of Trican have been detected in human breast milk from patients receiving Trican therapy; it should not be used by breastfeeding mothers.

Tell your doctor and pharmacist if you are allergic to Trican, other antifungal medications such as itraconazole (Sporanox), ketoconazole (Nizoral), or voriconazole (Vfend) or any other medications.

Do not take cisapride (Propulsid) while taking Trican.

Tell your doctor and pharmacist what prescription and nonprescription medications, vitamins, nutritional supplements, and herbal products you are taking, especially the following:

- Amiodarone (Cordarone)
- Anticoagulants (blood thinners) such as warfarin (Coumadin)
- Astemizole (Hismanal)
- Benzodiazepines such as midazolam (Versed)
- Cyclosporine (Neoral, Sandimmune)
- Disopyramide (Norpace)
- Diuretics (water pills) such as hydrochlorothiazide (HydroDIURIL, Microzide)
- Dofetilide (Tikosyn)
- Erythromycin (E.E.S, E-Mycin, Erythrocin)
- Isoniazid (INH, Nydrazid)
- Moxifloxacin (Avelox)
- Oral contraceptives (birth control pills)
- Oral medicine for diabetes such as glipizide (Glucotrol), glyburide (Diabeta, Micronase, Glycron, others), and tolbutamide (Orinase)
- Phenytoin (Dilantin)
- Pimozide (Orap)
- Procainamide (Procanbid, Pronestyl)
- Quinidine (Quinidex)
- Rifabutin (Mycobutin)
- Rifampin (Rifadin, Rimactane)
- Sotalolol (Betapace)

- Sparfloxacin (Zagam)
- Tacrolimus (Prograf)
- Terfenadine (Seldane)
- Theophylline (TheoDur)
- Thioridazine (Mellaril)
- Valproic acid (Depakene, Depakote)
- Zidovudine (Retrovir)

Tell your doctor if you drink or have ever drunk large amounts of alcohol and if you have or have ever had cancer; acquired immunodeficiency syndrome (AIDS); an irregular heartbeat; or heart, kidney or liver disease.

Tell your doctor if you are pregnant, plan to become pregnant, or are breast-feeding. If you become pregnant while taking Trican, call your doctor.

Symptoms of overdose may include:

- ☠ Hallucinations (seeing things or hearing voices that do not exist)
- ☠ Extreme fear that others are trying to harm you

Vagistat

Vagistat is an antifungal medication. It prevents fungus from growing. It is used to treat vaginal Candida (yeast) infections.

Vagistat is a brand name for the drug Tioconazole.

Avoid using condoms, cervical caps, or vaginal contraceptive diaphragms for 3 days following treatment with Vagistat. Vagistat contains oils that can weaken latex rubber condoms, diaphragms, or cervical caps. This increases the chance of a condom breaking during sex. The rubber in a cervical cap or diaphragm can also break down faster and wear out sooner.

Vaginal medicines usually will come out of the vagina during treatment. To keep the medicine from getting on your clothing, wear a minipad or sanitary napkin. The use of tampons is not recommended since they may soak up the medicine. To help clear up the infection, wear freshly washed cotton, not synthetic, underwear.

Side effects experienced when taking Vagistat may include:

- ☠ Shortness of breath
- ☠ Closing of your throat
- ☠ Swelling of your lips, face, or tongue
- ☠ Hives
- ☠ Burning
- ☠ Itching
- ☠ Irritation of the skin
- ☠ Increased need to urinate

Do not use Vagistat if you have a fever, abdominal pain, foul-smelling discharge, diabetes, HIV, or AIDS.

This means that it is not known whether Vagistat vaginal will be harmful to an unborn baby. Do not use this medication without first talking to your doctor if you are pregnant or could become pregnant during treatment.

It is not known whether Vagistat passes into breast milk. Do not use Vagistat vaginal without first talking to your doctor if you are breast-feeding a baby.

Vfend

Vfend works by preventing fungi from producing a substance called ergosterol, which is a component of fungal cell membranes. The cell membranes of fungi are vital for their survival. They keep unwanted substances from entering the cells and stop the contents of the cells from leaking out. Without ergosterol as part of the cell membrane, the membrane is weakened and damaged, and essential constituents of the fungal cells can leak out. This kills the fungi and hence clears up the infection.

Vfend is used to treat serious fungal infections, including those caused by Candida, Aspergillus, Scedosporium and Fusarium species of fungi. To make sure the fungi causing an infection are susceptible to Vfend your doctor may take a tissue sample, for example a swab from the throat or skin, or a urine or blood sample.

Vfend is usually reserved as treatment for progressive infections in people whose immune systems are under active, for example due to cancer treatment, AIDS, or following an organ transplant. Serious fungal infections can sometimes be life-threatening in these groups of patients.

Vfend is a brand name for the generic drug Voriconazole.

Before starting treatment with this medicine you should have a blood test to measure the levels of electrolytes (salts, such as potassium, calcium and magnesium) in your blood. If there are any problems your doctor will give you treatment to correct them before you start this medicine.

This medicine may cause visual disturbances such as blurred vision and so may affect your ability to drive or operate machinery safely. Do not drive or operate machinery until you know how this medicine affects you.

This medicine can make your skin more sensitive to sunlight. For this reason you should avoid exposing your skin to direct sunlight or sun lamps during treatment. Tell your doctor if you get a rash while taking this medicine.

This medicine can sometimes cause liver problems and for this reason your liver function will be monitored during treatment. Tell your doctor if you experience any of the following symptoms while taking this medicine, as they may suggest a problem with your liver:

- Unexplained itching
- Loss of appetite
- Nausea and vomiting
- Abdominal pain
- Yellowing of the skin or whites of the eyes (jaundice)
- Unusually dark urine or pale stools
- Your kidney function should also be monitored during treatment with this medicine.
- Unless your doctor tells you otherwise, it is important that you finish the prescribed course of this antifungal medicine, even if you feel better or it seems the infection has cleared up. Stopping the course early increases the chance that the infection will come back and that the fungi will grow resistant to the medicine.
- The following are some of the side effects that are known to be associated with this medicine:
- Visual disturbances.
- Fever
- Skin reactions such as rash or itch
- Disturbances of the gut such as diarrhea, constipation, nausea, vomiting or
- Abdominal pain.

- ☠ Headache
- ☠ Swelling of the legs and ankles due to fluid retention (peripheral edema)
- ☠ Flushing and nausea during infusion.
- ☠ Weakness
- ☠ Chest or back pain
- ☠ Respiratory distress syndrome
- ☠ Hair loss
- ☠ Low blood pressure
- ☠ Dizziness
- ☠ Hallucinations
- ☠ Confusion
- ☠ Depression
- ☠ Anxiety
- ☠ Tremor
- ☠ Pins and needles sensations
- ☠ Liver or kidney disorders
- ☠ Disturbances in the components of the blood
- ☠ Abnormal heart beats
- ☠ Inflammation of the pancreas (pancreatitis) in children

Vfend must not be used in combination with any of the following medicines:

- Astemizole
- Carbamazepine
- Cisapride
- Dihydroergotamine
- Ergotamine
- Phenobarbital

- Pimozide
- Quinidine
- Rifampicin
- High doses of ritonavir (400 mg and above twice daily)
- Sirolimus
- Terfenadine
- The herbal remedy St John's wort (Hypericum perforatum).

Vfend should be avoided in people taking low dose ritonavir (100 mg twice daily), unless your doctor considers the benefits to outweigh the risks. This is because ritonavir decreases the blood level of Vfend and could make it less effective at treating infection.

Vfend may increase the blood level of the immunosuppressants cyclosporine and tacrolimus. If you are taking cyclosporine or tacrolimus when you start this medicine your doctor should decrease your dose to prevent side effects from the immunosuppressant. The level of cyclosporine or tacrolimus in your blood should be monitored after starting and stopping treatment with this medicine.

Vfend may increase the anti-blood-clotting effect of anticoagulants such as warfarin. If you are taking an anticoagulant medicine your blood clotting time (INR) should be monitored while taking this medicine.

Vfend may increase the blood level of sulphonylurea medicines, such as tolbutamide, glipizide, glyburide, that are used to treat type 2 diabetes. This could cause blood sugar to fall (hypoglycemia). People taking any of these medicines should therefore carefully monitor their blood sugar during treatment with this medicine.

Vfend may increase the blood level of methadone. If you are taking methadone when you start this medicine your doctor may need to reduce your methadone dose in order to avoid side effects.

Vfend may increase the blood level of hormones from oral contraceptives containing ethinylestradiol and norethisterone. It should not make these contraceptives any less effective, but may increase the chance of getting side effects like nausea or changes in your bleeding.

Vfend may also increase the blood levels of the following medicines. As this could increase the chance of their side effects, your doctor may need to reduce the dose of these medicines if you are taking any of them when you start treatment with Vfend:

- Benzodiazepines such as Triazolam and midazolam
- Statins such as simvastatin
- Vincristine
- Vinblastine
- Omeprazole

Phenytoin and Rifabutin decrease the blood level of Vfend. Conversely, Vfend may increase the blood levels of these medicines. These combinations should be avoided where possible, but if considered necessary your doctor will prescribe you a higher than normal dose of Vfend and monitor you for side effects of the other medicine.

The anti-HIV medicine efavirenz also decreases the blood level of Vfend, while its blood level is increased by the Vfend. As a result, if you are taking efavirenz you will be prescribed a higher than normal dose of Vfend. In addition, your dose of efavirenz will be decreased during the treatment and then increased again once your course of Vfend is finished.

If you are taking other anti-HIV medicines, such as protease inhibitors, your doctor will want to monitor you carefully for any new side effects if you are also prescribed this medicine.

There may be an increased risk of abnormal heart rhythms (prolonged QT interval on the heart monitoring trace or ECG) if this medicine is taken with the following:

- Medicines to treat abnormal heart rhythms, eg amiodarone, procainamide, disopyramide, sotalol
- Certain antidepressants, such as maprotiline, amitriptyline, imipramine
- Certain antipsychotics, such as thioridazine, chlorpromazine, sertindole, haloperidol
- Antimalarials, such as halofantrine, chloroquine, quinine, Riamet
- Certain antimicrobials, eg erythromycin, moxifloxacin or pentamidine.

Vfend may cause harm to the fetus. Do not become pregnant while you are using it. If you think you may be pregnant, contact your doctor. You will need to discuss the benefits and risks of using Vfend while you are pregnant. It is not known if Vfend is found in breast milk. If you are or will be breast-feeding while you use Vfend, check with your doctor. Discuss any possible risks to your baby.

Voriconazole

Voriconazole works by preventing fungi from producing a substance called ergosterol, which is a component of fungal cell membranes. The cell membranes of fungi are vital for their survival. They keep unwanted substances from entering the cells and stop the contents of the cells from leaking out. Without ergosterol as part of the cell membrane, the membrane is weakened and damaged, and essential constituents of the fungal cells can leak out. This kills the fungi and hence clears up the infection.

Voriconazole is used to treat serious fungal infections, including those caused by Candida, Aspergillus, Scedosporium and Fusarium species of fungi. To make sure the fungi causing an infection are susceptible to voriconazole your doctor may take a tissue sample, for example a swab from the throat or skin, or a urine or blood sample.

Voriconazole is usually reserved as treatment for progressive infections in people whose immune systems are under active, for example due to cancer treatment, AIDS, or following an organ transplant. Serious fungal infections can sometimes be life-threatening in these groups of patients.

Voriconazole is sold under the brand name Vfend.

Before starting treatment with this medicine you should have a blood test to measure the levels of electrolytes (salts, such as potassium, calcium and magnesium) in your blood. If there are any problems your doctor will give you treatment to correct them before you start this medicine.

This medicine may cause visual disturbances such as blurred vision and so may affect your ability to drive or operate machinery safely. Do not drive or operate machinery until you know how this medicine affects you.

This medicine can make your skin more sensitive to sunlight. For this reason you should avoid exposing your skin to direct sunlight or sun lamps during treatment. Tell your doctor if you get a rash while taking this medicine.

This medicine can sometimes cause liver problems and for this reason your liver function will be monitored during treatment. Tell your doctor if you experience any of the following symptoms while taking this medicine, as they may suggest a problem with your liver:

- Unexplained itching
- Loss of appetite
- Nausea and vomiting
- Abdominal pain
- Yellowing of the skin or whites of the eyes (jaundice)
- Unusually dark urine or pale stools

Your kidney function should also be monitored during treatment with this medicine.

Unless your doctor tells you otherwise, it is important that you finish the prescribed course of this antifungal medicine, even if you feel better or it seems the infection has cleared up. Stopping the course early increases the chance that the infection will come back and that the fungi will grow resistant to the medicine.

The following are some of the side effects that are known to be associated with this medicine:

- Visual disturbances.
- Fever
- Skin reactions such as rash or itch

- ☠ Disturbances of the gut such as diarrhea, constipation, nausea, vomiting or abdominal pain.
- ☠ Headache
- ☠ Swelling of the legs and ankles due to fluid retention (peripheral edema)
- ☠ Flushing and nausea during infusion.
- ☠ Weakness
- ☠ Chest or back pain
- ☠ Respiratory distress syndrome
- ☠ Hair loss
- ☠ Low blood pressure
- ☠ Dizziness
- ☠ Hallucinations
- ☠ Confusion
- ☠ Depression
- ☠ Anxiety
- ☠ Tremor
- ☠ Pins and needles sensations
- ☠ Liver or kidney disorders
- ☠ Disturbances in the components of the blood
- ☠ Abnormal heart beats
- ☠ Inflammation of the pancreas (pancreatitis) in children

Voriconazole must not be used in combination with any of the following medicines:

- Astemizole
- Carbamazepine

- Cisapride
- Dihydroergotamine
- Ergotamine
- Phenobarbital
- Pimozide
- Quinidine
- Rifampicin
- High doses of ritonavir (400 mg and above twice daily)
- Sirolimus
- Terfenadine
- The herbal remedy St John's wort (Hypericum perforatum).

Voriconazole should be avoided in people taking low dose ritonavir (100 mg twice daily), unless your doctor considers the benefits to outweigh the risks. This is because ritonavir decreases the blood level of voriconazole and could make it less effective at treating infection.

Voriconazole may increase the blood level of the immunosuppressants cyclosporine and tacrolimus. If you are taking cyclosporine or tacrolimus when you start this medicine your doctor should decrease your dose to prevent side effects from the immunosuppressant. The level of cyclosporine or tacrolimus in your blood should be monitored after starting and stopping treatment with this medicine.

Voriconazole may increase the anti-blood-clotting effect of anticoagulants such as warfarin. If you are taking an anticoagulant medicine your blood clotting time (INR) should be monitored while taking this medicine.

Voriconazole may increase the blood level of sulphonylurea medicines, such as tolbutamide, glipizide, glyburide, that are used to treat type 2 diabetes. This could cause blood sugar to fall (hypoglycemia). People taking any of these medicines should therefore carefully monitor their blood sugar during treatment with this medicine.

Voriconazole may increase the blood level of methadone. If you are taking methadone when you start this medicine your doctor may need to reduce your methadone dose in order to avoid side effects.

Voriconazole may increase the blood level of hormones from oral contraceptives containing ethinylestradiol and norethisterone. It should not make these contraceptives any less effective, but may increase the chance of getting side effects like nausea or changes in your bleeding.

Voriconazole may also increase the blood levels of the following medicines. As this could increase the chance of their side effects, your doctor may need to reduce the dose of these medicines if you are taking any of them when you start treatment with Voriconazole:

- Benzodiazepines such as Triazolam and midazolam
- Statins such as simvastatin
- Vincristine
- Vinblastine
- Omeprazole

Phenytoin and Rifabutin decrease the blood level of Voriconazole. Conversely, Voriconazole may increase the blood levels of these medicines. These combinations should be avoided where possible, but if considered necessary your doctor will prescribe you a higher than normal dose of Voriconazole and monitor you for side effects of the other medicine.

The anti-HIV medicine efavirenz also decreases the blood level of Voriconazole, while its blood level is increased by the Voriconazole. As a result, if you are taking efavirenz you will be prescribed a higher than normal dose of Voriconazole. In addition, your dose of efavirenz will be decreased during the treatment and then increased again once your course of Voriconazole is finished.

If you are taking other anti-HIV medicines, such as protease inhibitors, your doctor will want to monitor you carefully for any new side effects if you are also prescribed this medicine.

There may be an increased risk of abnormal heart rhythms (prolonged QT interval on the heart monitoring trace or ECG) if this medicine is taken with the following:

- Medicines to treat abnormal heart rhythms, eg amiodarone, procainamide, disopyramide, sotalol
- Certain antidepressants, such as maprotiline, amitriptyline, imipramine
- Certain antipsychotics, such as thioridazine, chlorpromazine, sertindole, haloperidol
- Antimalarials, such as halofantrine, chloroquine, quinine, Riamet
- Certain antimicrobials, eg erythromycin, moxifloxacin or pentamidine.

Voriconazole may cause harm to the fetus. Do not become pregnant while you are using it. If you think you may be pregnant, contact your doctor. You will need to discuss the benefits and risks of using Voriconazole while you are pregnant. It is not known if Voriconazole is found in breast milk. If you are or will be breast-feeding while you use Voriconazole, check with your doctor. Discuss any possible risks to your baby.

Zeasorb

Zeasorb, an antifungal agent, is used for skin infections such as athlete's foot and jock itch and for vaginal yeast infections.

Zeasorb is a brand name for the generic drug Miconazole.

Zeasorb vaginal cream and suppositories are for use only in the vagina. These products are not to be taken by mouth. The vaginal suppositories are inserted, one per dose, in an applicator. Alternatively, the tube containing the vaginal cream is screwed onto the end of a special applicator tube, and the tube is then squeezed to fill the applicator. The patient then lies on her back with bent knees, inserts the applicator containing either the suppository or cream so that the tip of the applicator is high in the vagina, and then pushes the plunger in to deposit the suppository or cream into the vagina. The applicator should be washed with warm soap and water after each use.

Zeasorb usually is used once daily at bedtime. The 200 mg suppositories (Monistat 3) are inserted once nightly for 3 nights. The 100 mg suppositories

(Monistat-7) and intravaginal cream are inserted once nightly for 7 nights. The 1200 mg formulation (Monistat 1) is applied once for one night.

For fungal skin infections, the topical cream is applied as a thin layer to cover the affected skin and surrounding area, usually twice daily. The hands should be washed before and after application.

Zeasorb may cause the following side effects:

- Rash
- Burning at the site of application
- Itching
- Irritation of the skin or vagina
- Stomach pain
- Fever
- Foul-smelling vaginal discharge
- Diarrhea
- Vomiting
- Loss of appetite
- Hives
- Chills

There is very limited information on the use of Zeasorb during pregnancy. The physician must weigh the potential benefits against possible but unknown risks to the fetus.

It is not known if Zeasorb is secreted in breast milk in amounts that can affect the infant.

Tell your doctor about all the medicines you use (both prescription and nonprescription). Inform your doctor if you are taking:

- Anticoagulants (such as warfarin)
- Diabetes drugs
- Isoniazid
- Rifampin
- Rifabutin
- Phenytoin
- Cisapride

Made in the USA